THE NEW DASH DIET COOKBOOK 2021

How to induce Weight Loss and Improve Your Health with Delicious Meals

Contents

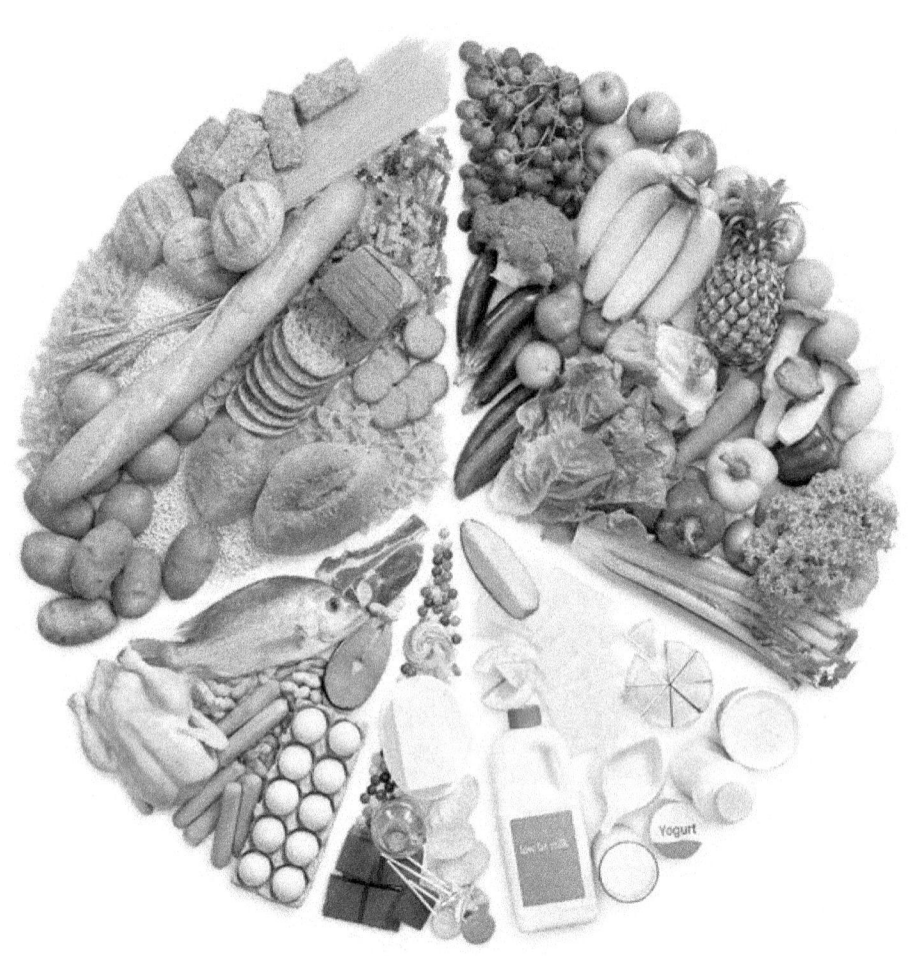

INTRODUCTIONS

High blood pressure is a severe health problem that affects more than a billion people around the world; and that number is rising every day. The number of people with high blood pressure has increased in the last decades. Hypertension is connected to a higher risk of conditions such as kidney failure, heart disease and stroke. DASH diet is thought to play a major role in the improvement of high blood pressure; scientists, medical personnel and policymakers have drafted specific dietary strategies to help reduce that number. DASH is an abbreviation for Dietary Approaches to bring Hypertension to an end. It is an eating plan that is based on recent research studies powered by the National Lung, Heart and Blood Institute. These recent researches showed that the DASH diet reduces and helps hypertension, while improving the level of cholesterol. This reduces your risk of having heart disease and other related illnesses. This book examines the DASH diet wholesomely, which was made to combat hypertension and reduce individual's risk of heart disease and other related ailment.

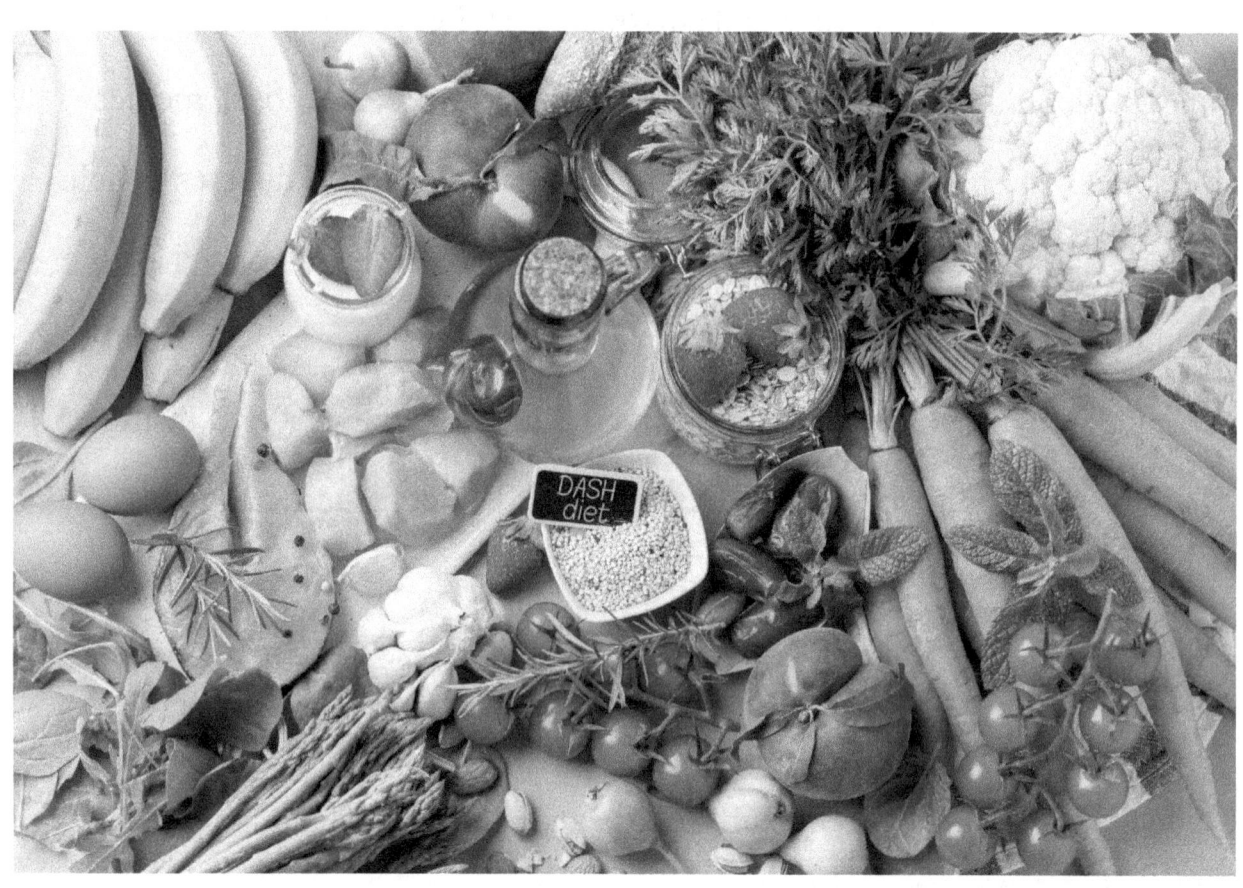

CHAPTER 1 - UNDERSTANDING THE DASH DIET

The DASH Diet (Dietary Approached to Stop Hypertension) is an admirable move by doctors to discover a way to stop hypertension, through the correct eating plan. It is an eating habit designed to bring down hypertension naturally. The DASH Diet is a diet that reduces one's intake of sodium. The diet allows the eating of fruits and vegetables, whole grain, fish and poultry, as well as nuts for snacks. The diet is high in magnesium, fiber, magnesium, calcium and potassium, which are important for good health. The dash diet usually focuses on keeping one's blood pressure below 120/80 mmHg.

Though the DASH Diet is not technically considered a vegetarian diet, it encourages the eating of fruits, nuts, vegetables and beans more than meats. All processed foods and junk food are not allowed in this diet at all. DASH diet allows all of the following:

- A lot of vegetables, fruits and fat-free or low-fat dairy
- Whole grains, beans, nuts and vegetable oils
- Encourages lean meats, poultry and fish
- Minimize the intake of salt, red meat, sweets and sugary drinks
- Minimize the intake alcoholic beverages

While on the DASH diet, you get to eat foods from all food compounds. But more of the foods that are usually low in salt, cholesterol and saturated fats should be added. Foods that are very rich in potassium, magnesium, calcium and fiber should also be involved. Below is a list of foods and how each should be eaten. For a diet that has over 3000 calories per day, you should eat:

- Vegetables (5 servings daily)
- Fruits (4 servings a daily)
- Skim or fat-free dairy products, like: milk and yogurt (2 to 3 servings a daily)
- Grains (6 to 8 servings daily - should be whole grains
- Fish, lean meats and poultry (2 servings or less a daily)
- Fats and oils (3 servings daily)

The diet has the ability to reduce the systolic blood pressure by 6 mm Hg. One's diastolic blood pressure by 3 mm Hg, is also given to reduce in dieters with normal blood pressure. With hypertension, scientists have been called to drop from 11 to 6 with the diet. It is also concluded that the utilization of the diet, in time, will reduce the risk of strokes and heart problems. So now, not only does hypertension ailments correct with the use of the DASH Diet, but it also has lots of benefits beyond what anyone ever imagined.

DASH diet recommendations:

- Little cholesterol and saturated fat

- Very low in sodium

- Very high in potassium, magnesium, calcium, protein and fiber

- Recommends fruits, vegetables and low-fat dairy

- Allows whole grains, fish, poultry and nuts

- Reduces red meat, sweets and sugary beverages

Points to Note

Following the DASH diet is very convenient and takes little time in the choice and preparation of food. Foods high in saturated fats and cholesterol should be tolerated. The individual involved is advised to eat many vegetables, fruits and cereals, as much as possible.

- As the foods you eat in a DASH Diet are rich in fiber content, it is concluded that in step-by-step increments, the consumption of fiber-rich food should be limited; to avoid the looseness of bowels and other stomach related diseases. You can little be little increment your fiber intake by eating an extra serving of leafy foods in each meals.

- Grains are another great wellsprings of fiber, just as B-complex vitamins and minerals. Entire grains, entire wheat bread, bran, wheat germ and low-fat breakfast cereals are a portion of the grain foods that you can eat, to build your fiber consumption.

- You can pick the meal you eat by taking a gander at the product labels of prepared and bundled foods. Search for foods that are low in fat, immersed fat, sodium and cholesterol. Meats, chocolates, chips and quick foods are the principle wellsprings of fat and cholesterol, so you ought to eliminate your consumption of these foods.

- If you want to eat meat, reduce your consumption to just six ounces per day, which is comparable in size to a deck of cards. You can also eat more vegetables, cereals, pasta and beans in your meat dishes. Low-fat milk or skim milk is also a quality source of protein without excess fat and cholesterol. You can go for canned or dried fruits, as well as fresh ones, instead of snacks.

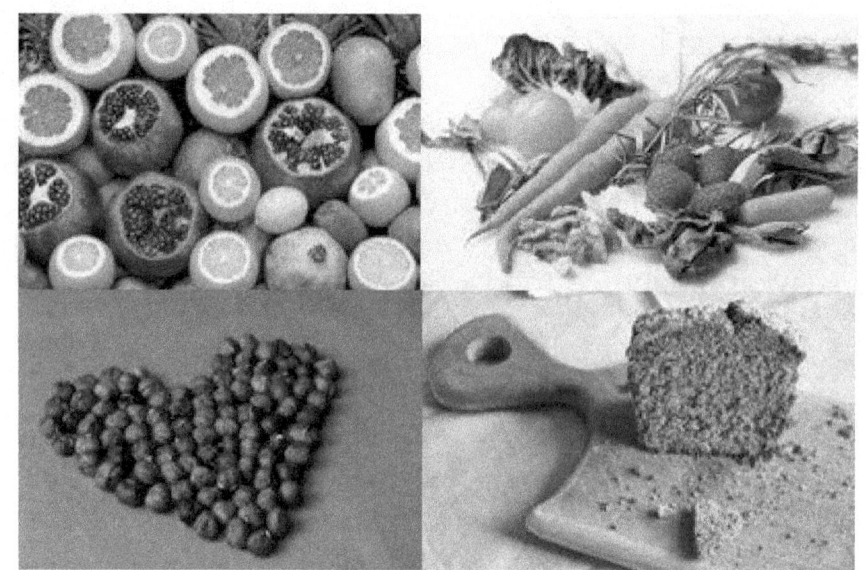

CHAPTER 2 - DASH DIET AND CHOLESTEROL

The fact that most people are experiencing cardiovascular problems and other related illnesses, due to increased blood cholesterol levels, illustrates the importance of balancing cholesterol levels in the body. Along with prescription drugs and regular exercise, following a DASH Diet regime seems to be the right alternative in reducing blood cholesterol.

It is essential to maintain healthy cholesterol levels for health and vitality. High amounts of cholesterol can cause a variety of diseases and conditions like hypertension, heart attacks and strokes. Cholesterol is found in foods like eggs, dairy products, fish, meat and poultry. Be aware of foods containing both high in saturated fat and cholesterol, such as dairy products; especially egg yolks and red meats.

The DASH diet can help in reducing cholesterol and blood pressure levels, which are the prime explanation behind the advancement of heart problems and sicknesses. It merits checking out because it can leave you feeling lighter, while giving you a more advantageous way of eating. You will get every one of the vegetables, low-fat dairy and natural products you need without feeling denied at any stage. You will be required to cut down on the amount of salt you consistently have with your nourishments. Salts can cause the development of liquids inside your body. This can, thus, put pressure on the heart. On the off chance that you choose to embrace the DASH approach, you will be required to cut down your utilization of salt to 2300 mg or lower. This again relies on your restorative history, race and age. However, it is a decent way to enable your heart to remain better. Get a lot of entire grains like bread produced using whole wheat, entire wheat pasta and cereal. Popcorn is a decent wellspring of fiber, which helps in bringing down cholesterol, and keeps you feeling full more. Breaking points your admission of calories to around 2000 every day by having six to seven little dinners. Remember to incorporate natural products alongside your diet, since they also can go far in assisting with such issues. Red wine is known to be loaded with resveratrol, a segment that is useful for the soundness of the heart. Do not be under the impression that you will be able to get the benefits of resveratrol by merely having a glass of red wine a day. For maximum benefits, you will be to consume at least 16 bottles of red wine, which will not only be impossible, but can also prove harmful. However, there is no reason for you to avoid giving your body the resveratrol it needs because today, you will not have any difficulties in finding resveratrol supplements, which also serve the same purpose. Include resveratrol supplements with a diet like DASH, and you will be well on your way to live life without heart problems.

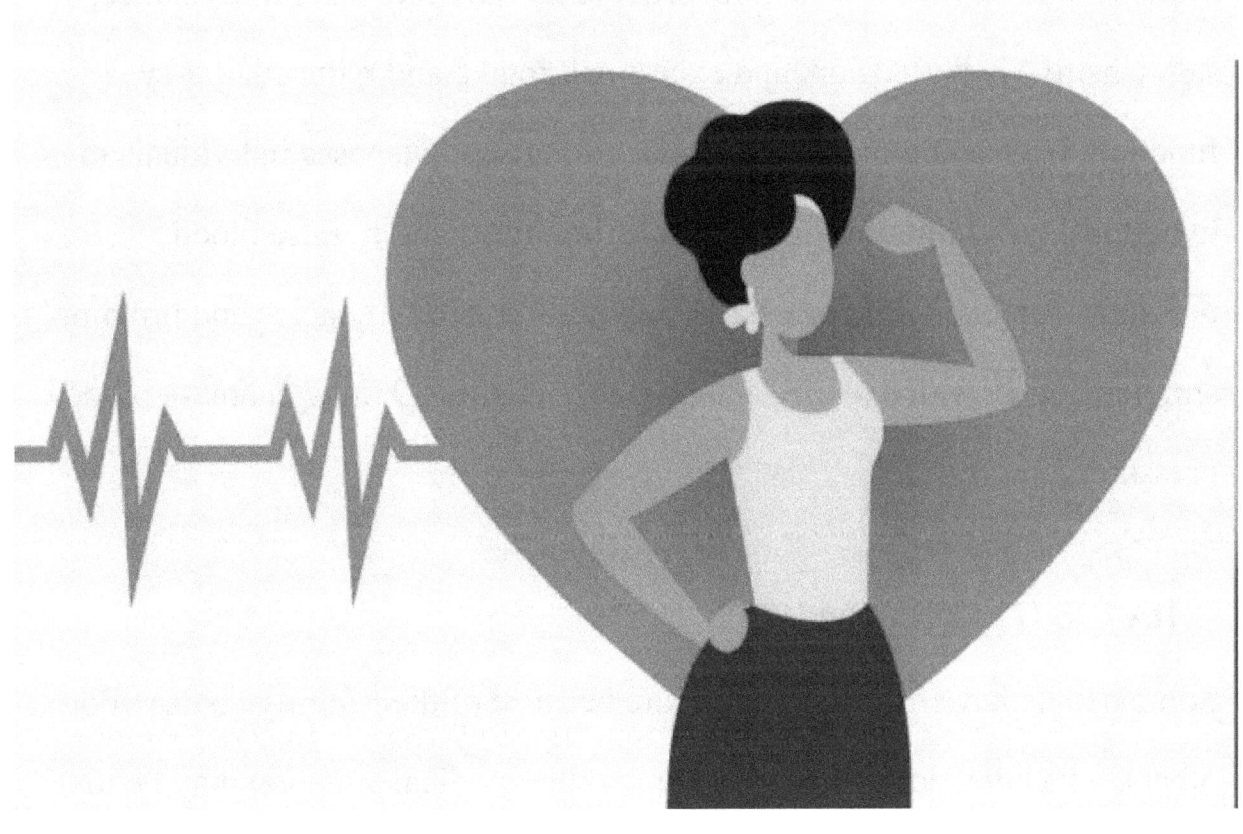

CHAPTER 3 - HOW NUTRITION AFFECTS HYPERTENSION (HIGH BLOOD PRESSURE)

The incidence and flinty nature of hypertension are affected by nutritional status and intake of many nutrients. Excessive energy intake and obesity are the core causes of hypertension. Obesity is associated with the increased activity of the renin-angiotensin-aldosterone and sympathetic nervous systems, possibly other mineralocorticoid activity like insulin resistance, salt-sensitive hypertension, and excess salt intake and reduced kidney function. High sodium chloride intake strongly predisposes individuals to hypertension. Continuous intake of alcohol may acutely raise blood pressure. Top eating of potassium, polyunsaturated fatty acids and protein, simultaneously with exercise and probably vitamin D, may decrease blood pressure.

WHAT IS HYPERTENSION?

Some people have high blood pressure because of their family history. For others, a bad diet, lack of exercise or another medical situation may be to blame. People who have high blood pressure always take medication. However, diet and exercise can help lower high blood pressure, even if it is a portion of your family history. High blood pressure fixes the heart in a way that it operates extra hard to pump nutrient and oxygen-rich blood to the body. The arteries that carry out the blood become weakened and less elastic. However, these changes happen to everyone as they become old; they happen more quickly in individuals with high hypertension. As the veins harden, the heart needs to work more earnestly, making the heart muscle thicker, more fragile, and less ready to pump blood adequately. At the point when high blood pressure harms the veins, they are not prepared to supply enough blood to organs for their legitimate working. Thus, body organs may get damaged, as well. For instance, this kind of harm can influence the heart, causing respiratory failure, affecting the cerebrum, causing a stroke, and the kidneys, promoting kidney disappointment.

High blood pressure is likewise known as hypertension. It can prompt extreme wellbeing confusion, and increase the danger of coronary illness, stroke and death. Hypertension is an essential hazard factor for cardiovascular sickness, including stroke, coronary failure, heart failure, aneurysm and related infirmity. Monitoring blood pressure is indispensable for safeguarding the wellbeing, and decreasing the dangers, of these risky conditions.

Hypertension is a common condition in which the constant force of the blood against your artery walls, are high enough that it may eventually lead to health problems, such as heart attack and diseases. Mainly the number of blood pumps of the heart, and the amount of resistance to blood flow in your arteries ascertains blood pressure. The higher amount of blood the heart pumps and tenses your arteries, the more increased the blood pressure is regularly. There are 2 phases of high blood pressure.

The primary hypertension phase: When the cause of high blood pressure is unknown. This is the most common phase of hypertension. This phase of blood pressure usually takes many years to develop. It probably is a result of one's lifestyle, habitat and how your body changes as we grow.

The hypertension phase: When a health problem or medicine is causing your high blood pressure. Things that can cause secondary hypertension phase include:

- Kidney predicaments and failures

- Obstructive sleep apnea

- Adrenal gland problems, etc.

- Congenital disabilities and challenges in the bloodstream

- Specific prescriptions, such as birth control tablets, cold remedies, decongestants, over-the-counter pain relievers and some prescription drugs

- Illegal drugs, such as cocaine and amphetamines

The increased pressure on your artery walls brought about by high blood pressure can harm your blood vessels, just as organs in your body. The more your blood pressure increases, and the more it goes uncontrolled, the more harmful the harm. Uncontrolled blood pressure can prompt entanglements, can include: weakening and narrowing blood vessels in your kidneys. Higher Pumping pressure of the blood by the heart against the higher pressure in the blood vessels, this causes the arteries of the heart's siphoning chamber to thicken (left ventricular hypertrophy). Inevitably, the thickened muscle may make some hard memories siphoning enough blood to address your body's tissues, which can prompt cardiovascular breakdown and issue

Uncontrolled high blood pressure affects your capability to think, remembering things and learns. The problem of memory loss or forgetfulness is more common in individuals with high blood pressure. Weakened or blocked arteries can limit blood flow to the brain, leading to a particular type of dementia called vascular dementia. A stroke or ailment that interrupts blood flow to the brain also can cause vascular dementia and related issues.

High blood pressure can also cause solidifying and thickening of the arteries (atherosclerosis), which can prompt a coronary failure, stroke or various confusions.

Increased blood pressure can make your blood vessels debilitate and swell, framing an aneurysm. On the off chance that an aneurysm breaks, it tends to be perilous.

Controlling and maintaining your high blood pressure is a lifelong adhesion. You will always need to watch your weight, make healthy food choices, exercise, learn to manage and cope with stress, eschew smoking and limit your alcohol intake. If medicine is needed to control your high blood pressure, you will likely need it all your life. Additionally, it is essential to cultivate the attitude of regular blood pressure checks. Your doctor may want you to come to the hospital regularly.

Blood pressure can be injurious regardless of whether it remains just marginally over the ordinary degree of 120/80 mmHg. The more your blood pressure transcends typical, the more hazardous to your wellbeing. Researchers upheld by the National Heart, Lung and Blood Institute (NHLBI) led two key investigations. Their findings demonstrated that blood pressures were reduced with an eating plan that is low in immersed fat, cholesterol, all-out fat and that underscores natural products, vegetables; without fat or low-fat milk and milk products.

The DASH eating plan additionally incorporates entire grain products, fish and fish products, poultry and nuts. DASH diet is reduced in lean and red meat, desserts, included sugars, and sugar-containing refreshments and beverages contrasted with the regular American diet. It is wealthy in potassium, magnesium and calcium, just as protein and fiber.

The DASH eating plan follows heart-sound guidelines to confine soaked fat and cholesterol. It centers on expanding the admission of foods wealthy in supplements that are required to lower blood pressure, for the most part, minerals like potassium, magnesium and calcium, protein and fiber. It incorporates supplement rich foods with the goal that it meets other supplement necessities, as suggested by the Institute of Medicine. The

DASH eating guide requires a specific number of day-by-day servings from different food gatherings. The measure of servings you require may differ contingent upon your caloric needs. The DASH eating guide, utilized alongside another way of life changes, can assist you with averting and control blood pressure. On the off chance that blood pressure isn't excessively high, you might have the option to control it completely just by changing your eating propensities and plan, shedding pounds if overweight, getting ordinary exercise and physical exercises and eliminating or shunning liquor. The DASH eating guide additionally has different advantages, for example, lowering terrible cholesterol, which, alongside lowering blood pressure, can lessen your danger of getting the coronary illness.

FOOD GROUP	SERVINGS	SERVING SIZE	EXAMPLES
vegetables	4-5 per day	1 cup raw leafy greens Half cup chopped cooked vegetables Half cup vegetable juice	low sodium tomato juice, Lettuce, kale, spinach, broccoli, carrots, green beans, squash, sweet potatoes, tomatoes, asparagus, green peppers,
Grains	4-7 per day	2 slice of bread	wheat bread and rolls, wheat

		Half cup cooked rice, pasta or grain	pasta, pita bread, quinoa, rice, popcorn, oatmeal, pretzels
Fruits	4-5 per day	1 medium fruit 1/4 cup of dried fruit 1/2 cup 100% fruit juice	peaches, pears, grapes, melons, raisins, dried apricots, apples, bananas, berries, oranges, pineapple
Non-Fat Milk and Dairy Products	2-4 per day	1 cup yogurt 1 1/2 ounce cheese	fat-free or low fat regular or frozen yogurt, non-fat milk, reduced fat cheese per day
Beans, Nuts, Seeds	4 per weekly	1 1/2 ounce nuts 2 tablespoons of peanut butter half ounce seeds Half cup of beans or peas	peanuts, peanut butter, kidney beans, pinto beans, lentils, split peas, Almonds, walnuts, sunflower seeds,
Poultry, Fish, Lean Meats	4-6 ounce per day	1 ounce prepare meat, poultry or fish meals 1 egg = 1-ounce serving	lean meat and trim off visible fat, remove the skin from poultry. Bake, broil or poach
Oils, Fats	2 per day	1 spoon soft margarine 1 spoon vegetable oil	margarine, vegetable oils (corn, olive or safflower), low-fat mayonnaise, light salad dressing

Desserts, Sweets, Added Sugars	4 or less per day	1 tablespoon jelly Half cup sorbet	Jams and jellies, fruit punch, candy, maple syrup, sorbet and ices, sugar

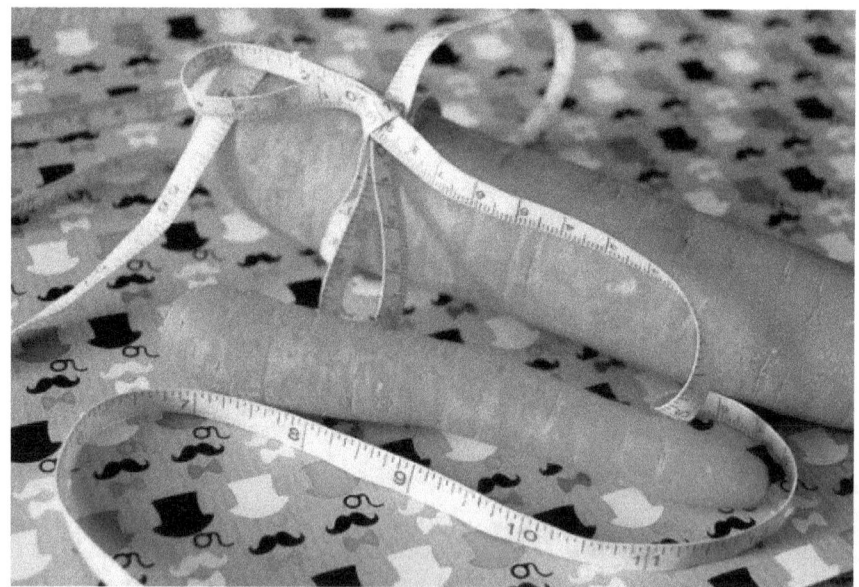

Go for fruit as your *easy to grab* snacks. Eat fruit that is ready to eat like apples, bananas, cucumber or canned cut fruit. Go for canned fruit that is canned in juice.

Try pasta and stir-fry dishes. They are good ways to eat less red meat and more

vegetables, beans and grains. Always put an additional vegetable serving to your meals, especially lunch and dinner. Prepare fresh vegetables and keep them in a clean and clear container in the fridge in your kitchen. This will make it faster for you when you want to use them.

Make it a habit. Keep frozen vegetables handy to add to casseroles and soups.

Choose whole-grain products whenever you can. This will help fill you up and add fiber

to your diet. Include low-fat milk in your meals. Replace sweetened drinks with low-fat milk. Gradually reduce your portion size of the meat, fish and poultry products. Fill your plate with more vegetables instead. Take low-fat yogurt or a little piece of low-fat cheese.

Take the salts off the table. Do not include salt when preparing your meals, or cut the amount to be added.

Processed foods should be avoided.

EXAMPLES OF FOOD GROUPS	SIGNIFICANCE OF EACH FOOD GROUP TO THE DASH DIETS EATING METHOD	
Muffin, bagel, cereals, rice, pita bread, oatmeal, unsalted pretzels and popcorn, Whole wheat bread and rolls, whole wheat pasta are allowed	The major sources of energy and fiber	
green beans, kale, lima beans, potatoes, spinach, broccoli, squash, sweet potatoes, tomatoes works fine	Rich source of magnesium, potassium, and fiber	
Apples, apricots, melons, bananas, dates, grapefruit, oranges, mangoes, pineapples, strawberries very good	Important sources of potassium, magnesium and fibre	
low-fat milk or buttermilk, fat-free, low-fat cheese, fat-free or low-fat regular or frozen yogurt are great	The main source of calcium and protein and many more	
kidney beans, lentils, split peas, almonds, hazelnuts, mixed nuts,	Full of fiber, magnesium, and protein	

peanuts, walnuts, sunflower seeds, peanut butter		

In case you're taking a shot at getting in shape, utilize the foods and serving rules in the table above. Focus on a caloric level that is lower than what you generally consume. Additionally, you can make your diet lower in calories by utilizing the tips. The most proper approach to take off pounds is to do so continuously, get progressively physical with activity, and eat a fair diet that is lower in calories and fat. For certain individuals at extremely high hazard for coronary illness or stroke, medicine will be fundamental. To build up a weight-misfortune or weight-support program that function admirably for you, counsel with your primary care physician or enlisted dietitian.

Joining the DASH eating plan with a normal physical activity program, for example, strolling or swimming, will help you both shed pounds and remain trim as long as possible. You can do an activity for 30 or more minutes one after another, or pick shorter times in any event, 10 minutes each. The basic thing is to aggregate around 30 minutes of activity every day.

You ought to know that the DASH eating plan has all the more day-by-day servings of fruits, vegetables and whole-grain foods than you might be accustomed to eating. Since the DASH diet plan is high in fiber, it can prompt swelling and the runs in certain people. To maintain a strategic distance from these issues, with step-by-step increments, increase your intake of fruit, vegetables and whole-grain foods. The key to diminishing salt intake is settling on astute food decisions and practice good eating habits. Just a little quantity of salt that we consume is from the salt included at the dining or eating table, and just limited quantities of sodium happen normally in food, it is encouraged to investigate food and product labels to pick products less in sodium. You might be shocked to know which foods contain sodium. This incorporates heated products, certain oats, soy sauce, prepared salts, monosodium glutamate, preparing pop and a few acid neutralizers; the range is wide.

Calories on the DASH Eating Guide

The DASH eating guide can be engaged to enhance weight loss. Because it is rich in lower-calorie foods, such as fruits and vegetables. You can reduce calorie intake by replacing higher calorie foods, such as sweets, with more fruits and vegetables, and that also will make it easier for you to reach your DASH goals. Here are some examples:

Increase Fruits Intake

- Eat a medium apple instead of bread and cookies. You'll save more than 80 calories.

- Eat one-quarter cup of dried apricots instead of a 2-ounce bag of pork rinds. You'll save 230 calories.

Increase Vegetables

- Take a hamburger that contains 3 ounces of meat instead of 6 ounces. Add a half-cup serving of carrots and a half-cup serving of spinach. You'll save more than 200 calories.

Increase Fat-free or Low-fat Milk Products

- Take a half-cup serving of low-fat frozen yogurt instead of a half-cup serving of full-fat ice cream. You'll save more than 70 calories.

Essential Calorie Saving Tips:

- Eat smaller portions of food

- Choose milk product free or low in fat

- Always check the food labels to compare fat content in packaged foods—items marked fat-free or low fat are not always lower in calories than their regular versions.

- Reduce intake foods with lots of added sugar, such as pies, flavored yogurts, candy bars, ice cream, sherbet, regular soft drinks and fruit drinks.

- Go for fruits canned in their own juice or in water.

- Always put the fruit to plain fat-free yogurt.

- Snack on natural products, vegetable sticks, unbuttered and unsalted popcorn, or rice cakes.

- Take water as is or with a wedge of lemon or lime.

Tips To Reduce Salt and Sodium in the DASH Diet Plan

- Go for reduced-sodium or no-salt-added versions of foods and condiments.

- Go for fresh, frozen or canned vegetables that are low-sodium or no-salt-added

- Use fresh poultry, fish and lean meat instead of canned, smoked or processed types.

- Go breakfast cereals that are lower in sodium.

- Reduce intake of cured foods, such as bacon

- Cook rice and other related cereals without salt.

- Choose foods that are lower in sodium. Reduce intake of frozen dinners, mixed dishes such as pizza, packaged mixes, canned soups or broths and salad dressings—these often have a lot of sodium.

- Rinse canned foods to wash away part of the sodium.

- Use spices instead of salt. In preparing at the table, flavor meals with herbs, spices, lemon, lime or salt-free seasoning blends. Start by reducing salt in half.

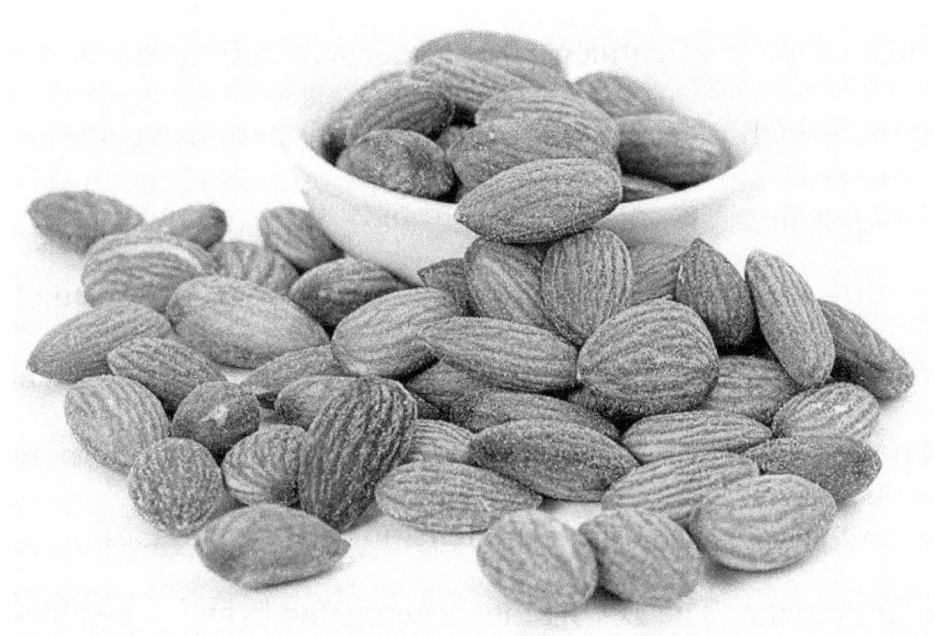

CHAPTER 6 - LIFESTYLE CHANGES/MODIFICATION AND HYPERTENSION

High Blood Pressure is one of the essential and familiar risk factors for atherosclerotic cardiovascular disease and renal disease. The contemporary approach to the prevalence of elevated Blood Pressure and its complications involves pharmacologic treatment of hypertensive individuals and "lifestyle modification," which is beneficial for both non-hypertensive and hypertensive persons. Recent research strongly supports the concept that lifestyle modification can have powerful effects on BP. Increased physical activity, reduced salt intake, weight loss, moderation of alcohol intake, increased potassium intake and an overall healthy dietary pattern, termed the Dietary Approaches to Stop Hypertension (DASH) diet, effectively lower Blood Pressure. The DASH diet accentuates fruits, vegetables and low or no-fat dairy products and is less in fat and cholesterol. Other dietary factors, such as a more intake of protein or monounsaturated fatty acids, may also reduce Blood pressure. The current issues with health care providers, researchers, government and the general public is bringing and issuing out effective clinical and public health strategies that bring to sustained lifestyle modification.

The move to bring down the epidemic of High Blood Pressure and its cardiovascular and renal complications has traditionally faced on the pharmacological treatment of persons with established hypertension. Such endeavors mirror an amazing collection of proof that has archived the useful impacts of antihypertensive medication treatment in averting Blood Pressure -related clinical intricacies. All things considered, dependence on sedate treatment alone is a deficient answer for the pandemic of high blood pressure and its difficulties. To begin with, it is very much perceived that the danger of Blood Pressure related cardiovascular and renal illness increments continuously all through the scope of Blood Pressure, including scopes of Blood Pressure recently thought to be ordinary. More also, a large number of adults have a BP that is above optimal, and yet is below the natural threshold for drug treatment. Such Blood Pressure levels are not to place individuals at increased risk of hypertension-related complications, yet they are not candidates for drug therapy. In lieu of these considerations, national and international law, making bodies recommend and suggest lifestyle modification as a means to prevent and treat hypertension and thereby prevent cardiovascular and renal disease in the whole population.

The DASH diet is known for its low saturated fat, red meat, sugar, sugary drinks and refined carbohydrates, but high in fruits, vegetables, whole grains, fish, poultry and low-fat dairy products. The DASH diet has been proven to reduce weight, heart rate, risk of type 2 diabetes, C reactive protein, Apolipoprotein B and homocysteine, and is associated with a lower issue of heart failure, all bring about mortality and stroke.

Recent studies discovered that the replacement of some of the DASH diet's carbohydrate intake with either protein (50% from plant sources) or unsaturated fat (mainly monounsaturated, found in olives and olive oil) could reduce blood pressure, low-density lipoprotein, homocysteine and coronary heart disease risk even further.

The DASH diet combined with reduced alcohol and salt intake, weight loss, physical activities and aerobic exercise achieved a reduction of 14.2/7.4 mmHg among hypertensive, and while hypertension prevalence fell over a period of 6 months from 38% to 12%. 15 Salt reduction, possibly the single most important hypertensive measure, involves staying away from processed foods, regularly checking food labels for salt content and using herbs or spices for flavor.

Lifestyle modification, previously appalled non-pharmacologic therapy, has important roles in hypertensive, as well as non-hypertensive individuals. In hypertensive individuals, lifestyle changes can serve as an initial treatment before the start of drug therapy and as an adjunct to medication in persons already on drug therapy. In hypertensive people through medication-controlled Blood Pressure, to some extent, these therapies can bring about drug step-down, and drug withdrawal in highly motivated people who achieve and sustain lifestyle changes. In people that are not hypertensive, lifestyle guild have the qualities to stop hypertension, and more largely, to reduce BP and thereby decrease the risk of BP-related clinical complications in whole populations. Indeed, even an ostensibly small reduction in Blood Pressure, if applied to an entire population, could have an enormously beneficial effect on cardiovascular events. For instance, a 3-mmHg stops in Systolic Blood Pressure should lead to an 8% reduction in stroke mortality, and a 5% reduction in mortality from coronary heart disease. Beware some highlights of specific lifestyle therapies that reduce hypertension.

Increasing Physical Activities

Increased level of physical activity and aerobic exercise lowers Blood Pressure drastically, irrespective of coexistent changes in weight. Blood Pressure among individuals assigned to an aerobic exercise and physical activity intervention has proven to be a good edge, as far as hypertension is concerned. The significance of Blood Pressure change appeared to be independent of the exercise intensity. In addition, increased physical activity should also lower Blood Pressure by facilitating initial weight loss, and by promoting maintenance of weight loss, once achieved.

Cut back on Salt (Sodium Chloride) Intake.

A high eating of salt, also known as sodium chloride, adversely causes some issues in hypertension. Evidence includes results from animal studies, epidemiologic studies and clinical trials. Decreasing the sodium intake can stop hypertension, can bring about hypertension control in older-aged persons on drugs and can potentially stop cardiovascular events in overweight individuals. Sodium chloride decrease, alone or combined with weight loss, can minimize the incidence of hypertension by approximately 20%, a reduced salt intake with or without weight loss effectively decrease Blood Pressure, and the need for antihypertensive drugs in older persons.

Tips to consider lessening sodium intake:

- Eat fewer processed foods. Only a small amount of sodium occurs normally in foods. Most sodium is added during preparation.

- Peruse food labels and descriptions, and go for low-sodium alternatives to the foods you normally buy.

- Don't add salt, but if at all, only do 1 teaspoon of salt, which represents 2,300 mg of sodium; use herbs or spices to add flavor to your food.

Moderating Alcohol Intake

The connection between high alcohol and liquor intake and hypertension has been reported in numerous epidemiologic investigations. Preliminaries have likewise announced that decreases in alcohol intake can bring down Blood Pressure in normotensive, and hypertensive men who are substantial consumers. A decrease in liquor admission brought Blood Pressure down to a little, non-critical degree. In total, the accessible proof backings a suggestion to restrain alcohol intake is to go for two bottles for every day (men), and one bottle for each day (ladies) among the individuals who drink.

Increase intake of Potassium. As opposed to the immediate relationship of salt intake with hypertension, elevated levels of potassium are related to low Blood Pressure. All things considered, an average portion of 60 to 120 mmol/d of supplemental potassium diminished systolic and diastolic Blood

Pressure by 4.4 and 2.5 mmHg in hypertensive people and by 1.8 and 1.0 mmHg in normotensives. High dietary intake of potassium can be accomplished through diet as opposed to pills, and in light of the fact that potassium got from foods additionally accompanies an assortment of different supplements; the favored technique to expand potassium admission is to devour foods wealthy in potassium, instead of enhancements. Increment potassium admission is significant for dealing with your circulatory strain and lessening your danger of heart assault, stroke and other wellbeing dangers.

Always read the labels

By soaking up the propensity for reading food labels, you can pick foods all the more shrewdly. Look out for foods that have saturated fat or Tran's fat before buying. With so many marketing messages being tossed at you in the supermarket and grocery store, it very well may be hard to tell what is genuinely sound. To make it simpler, the American Heart Association (AHA) built up the Heart-Check mark. At the point when you see this image on food packaging, it implies that the product meets AHA criteria for saturated fat, Trans fat and sodium for a solitary serving of the food product for sound individuals over age 2.

Eschew smoking and related habits

Every cigarette you smoke builds your circulatory strain for a long time after you finish. Halting smoking enables your blood to pressure to come back to typical. Stopping smoking can diminish your danger of coronary illness and improve your general wellbeing. Peoples who stop smoking may live longer than peoples who never stop smoking.

Cut back on caffeine intake

The part caffeine plays in blood pressure, is still being contemplated by medical personnel. It is capable of raising blood pressure up to 15 mm Hg in individuals who rarely consume it. Despite the fact that people who drink espresso normally may encounter next to zero impact on their blood pressure. Despite the fact that the long haul impacts of caffeine on circulatory strain aren't clear, it's conceivable that it may somewhat increase. To check whether caffeine raises your circulatory strain, check your weight inside 30 minutes of drinking charged refreshment. In any case that your pulse increments by 5 to 10 mm Hg, you might be delicate to the blood pressure raising impacts of caffeine. Converse with your primary care physician about the impacts of caffeine on your circulatory strain.

Reduce your stress

Constant stress may add to hypertension. More research is expected to decide the impacts of incessant stress on the pulse. Intermittent stress likewise can add to hypertension on the off chance that you respond to stress by eating undesirable nourishment, drinking liquor or smoking. Set aside some effort to consider what causes you to feel stressed, for example, work, family, accounts or ailment. When you comprehend what's causing your stress, think about how you can take out or diminish stress. In the event that you can't kill the entirety of your stressors, you can, at any rate, adapt to them in a more beneficial manner.

Try to:

- Pay more attention to issues you can control and make plans to determine them.

- Try to keep away from stress triggers and stressors when you can. For instance, if heavy traffic while in transit to work causes stress, take a stab at leaving prior toward the beginning of the day, or take open transportation. Stay away from individuals who cause you stress, if conceivable.

- Create time to relax and to do activities you enjoy. Require some investment every day to sit quietly and breathe deeply.

- Plan your day and focus on your needs. Abstain from attempting to do excessively and figure out how to say no in certain circumstances. Understand, there are a few things you can't change or control. However, you can focus on how you respond to them, and this goes far to help.

- Expressing appreciation to others can help decrease your stress.

Follow up your blood pressure

Self-monitoring can help you with watching your blood pressure and circulatory strain, make certain your lifestyle changes are working, and alert you and your doctor to potential wellbeing confusions. Monitor your blood pressure, generally with a prescription. Chat with your primary care physician about home monitoring before you start. Typical experiences with your primary care physician are key to controlling your blood pressure. To ensure that your circulatory strain is well-controlled, check with your primary care physician about how routinely you need to check it. Your primary care physician may prescribe checking it step-by-step or less consistently. In case you're not observing any improvements in your prescriptions or different treatments, your doctor may suggest you check your blood pressure beginning two weeks after treatment changes, and seven days before your next arrangement.

In addition to the emotional imbalance we feel when faced with a stressful situation, our bodies respond by releasing stress hormones, which are adrenaline and cortisol into the bloodstream. These hormones prepare the body for the by making the heart beat faster, and constricting blood vessels to get more blood to the core of the body instead of the extremities. Compaction of blood vessels can cause your heart rate to go high, does increase blood pressure, but only majorly when the stress reaction goes away, does the blood pressure returns to its pre-stress level. This is referred to as situational stress, and its effects are generally short-lived, and disappear when the stressful event is over.

Although our modern world has many stressful events that we can't handle those options. Chronic stress level causes our bodies to go into high gear on and off for days or weeks at a time. The relationship between chronic stress and blood pressure are not clear and are still being studied.

How Stress Affects Your Body

- Stress makes the adrenal organ discharge adrenaline into the body, which encourages your body to react to risk by expanding heart rate, contracting blood vessels and changing over fat to vitality. Your body additionally discharges cortisol during stress, which has many harming consequences for the body when unregulated. The expansion in hormones makes the liver produce more glucose and strains the body's capacity to reabsorb the sugar, causing diabetes. Stress can cause expanded and shallow breathing or holding of your breath, implying that cells don't get enough oxygen. This can prompt discombobulating, absence of fixation and transient lose cognizance.

- When you are under stress, your heart pulsates quicker, attempting to siphon blood rapidly around your body to prepare it for activity. Blood pressure is raised and when under stress, and it very well may be raised for a really long time, causing long haul problems for the body.

- Heartburn, indigestion, ulcers and esophageal fits are all medical problems that can be attached to stress in the body, as your body creates progressively corrosive and controls what supplements you assimilate during times of high stress. This can likewise cause a stoppage and the runs.

- During times of high stress, muscles are continually fixed, prompting torment, damage and incessant issues like headaches and pressure cerebral pains.

Lessening your feeling of anxiety and stress may not straightforwardly bring down your blood pressure over the long haul. Be that as it may, utilizing techniques to deal with your pressure can help improve your wellbeing in different manners. Mastering the stress management techniques and methods can prompt solid behavioral changes, including those that lessen your blood pressure. There are numerous alternatives for overseeing pressure.

For example:

- Relax.
- If you always feel rushed and tensed, take a few minutes to review your calendar and to-do lists. Check for activities that take up your time, but aren't very important to you. Schedule less time for these activities or eliminate them completely, and all this will help simplify your whole schedule.
- Number deep and slow breaths to help you relax.
- Physical activity is a natural stress buster. Just be sure to get your doctor's go-ahead before starting a new exercise program, especially if you've been diagnosed with high blood pressure.
- Yoga strengthens your body and helps relaxation. These techniques also may lower your systolic blood pressure by 6 millimeters of mercury (mm Hg) or more.

Participation in regular physical activity and aerobic exercise is a key modifiable determinant of hypertension and is recognized as a cornerstone therapy for the primary prevention, treatment, and control of high BP. On average, regular aerobic exercise decrease resting systolic Blood Pressure 5-7 mmHg, while preventing exercise decrease resting systolic Blood Pressure 2-3 mmHg within individuals with hypertension. Levels of physical activity and aerobics in modern urbanized society are not insufficient to keep up good health and to prevent cardiovascular and other diseases. Aerobic exercise is almost part of free of secondary effects, and is a useful prolongs therapy in treating hypertension. There are many possible mechanisms to account for the beneficial effects of exercise in bringing down the blood pressure, the bringing about physiological effects usually also classified as acute, post-exercise, or chronic. What is the connection between hypertension and physical activities? Regular physical activity and aerobics make your heart stronger and effective. A strong and healthy heart can pump more blood with less effort. If the heart can work less to pump blood, then the force and pressure on your arteries decrease, lowering your blood pressure.

Aerobic activity can be a viable method to control hypertension. In any case, adaptability and reinforcing activities, for example, lifting loads, are likewise significant pieces of a general fitness plan. You don't have to go through hours in the gym center each day to profit by aerobic activity. Essentially adding moderate physical exercises to your everyday schedule will help. Any physical activity that expands your heart, and breathing rates, are viewed as aerobic activity, including:

- Household chores, such as mowing, raking leaves, gardening or scrubbing the floor.
- Action sports, like basketball or tennis.
- Climbing stairs.
- Walking around the neighborhood.
- Jogging.
- Cycling.
- Swimming, dancing and drama activities.

CHAPTER 8 - DASH DIET BREATFAS RECIPES

1. Layered Hummus Dip

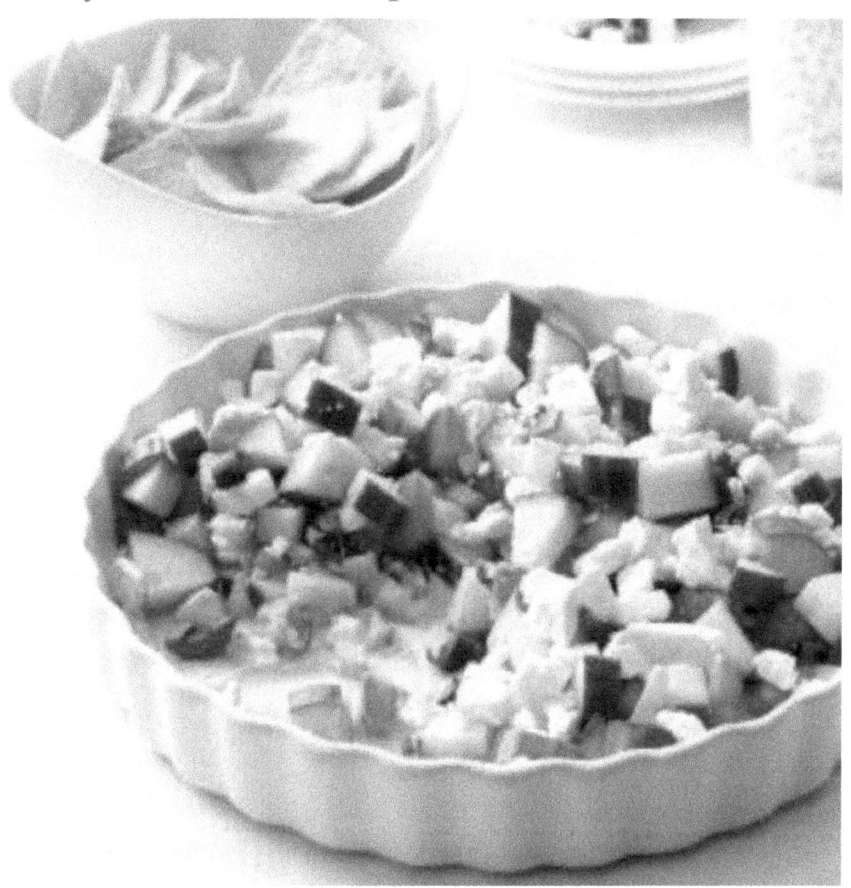

Prep Time: 15 mins

Total Time: 15 mins

Servings : 12

_____

Ingredients

- [ ] 1 carton (10 ounces) hummus
- [ ] 1/4 cup finely chopped red onion
- [ ] 1/2 cup Greek olives, chopped
- [ ] 2 medium tomatoes, chopped and seeded
- [ ] 1 English, large cucumber chopped
- [ ] 1 cup crumbled feta cheese
- [ ] Pita baked

Directions

1. Spread hummus into a shallow 10-in. round dish. Layer with onion, olives, tomatoes, cheese and cucumber. Refrigerate until serving. Serve with chips.

2. Warm Rice & Pintos Salad

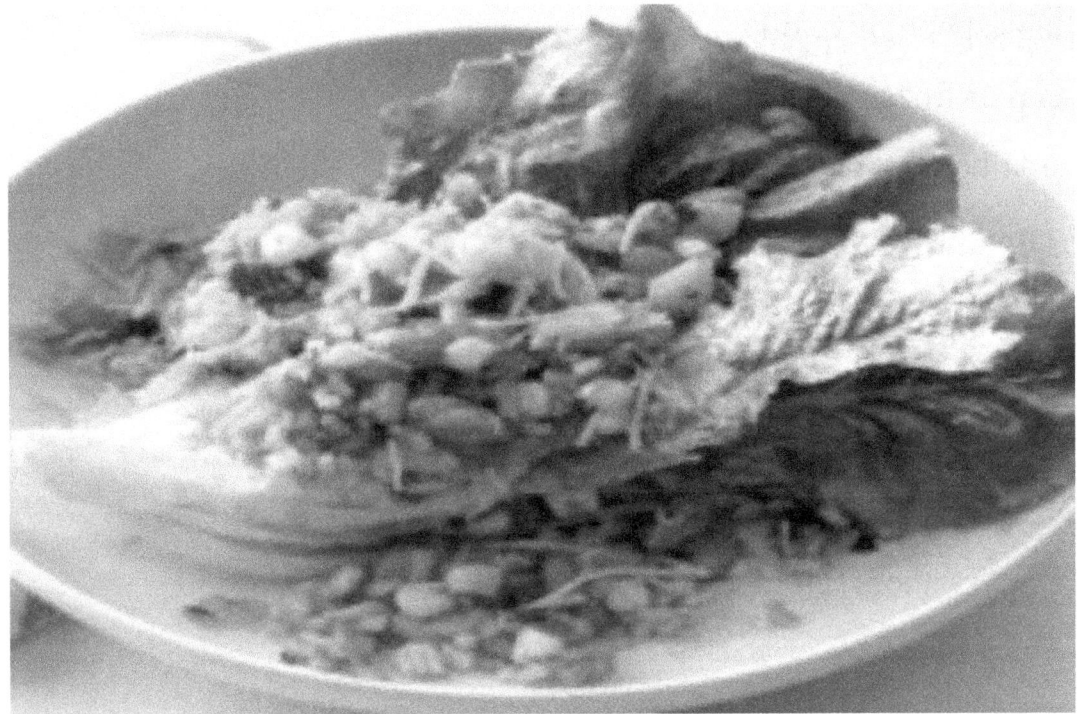

Prep Time: 10 mins

Cook Time: 20 mins

Total Time: 30 mins

Servings: 4

Ingredients

- ☐ 1 tablespoon olive oil
- ☐ 1 cup of frozen corn
- ☐ 1 small onion, chopped
- ☐ 2 garlic cloves, minced
- ☐ 1-1/2 teaspoons chilli powder
- ☐ 1-1/2 teaspoons ground cumin
- ☐ 1 can (15 ounces) pinto beans, rinsed and drained
- ☐ 1 package (8.8 ounces) ready-to-serve brown rice
- ☐ 1 can (4 ounces) chopped green chillies
- ☐ 1/2 cup salsa
- ☐ 1/4 cup chopped fresh cilantro
- ☐ 1 bunch romaine, quartered lengthwise through the core
- ☐ 1/4 cup finely shredded cheddar cheese

Directions

1. In a large bowl, preheat the oil over medium-high heat. Put together corn and onion; boil and stir 4-5 minutes or until onion is soft. Stir in garlic, chilli powder and cumin; cook and stir 1 minute longer.

2. Add beans, rice, green chillies, salsa and cilantro; heat through, stirring occasionally.

3. Serve over romaine wedges. Sprinkle with cheese.

3. Barbecued Basil Turkey Burgers

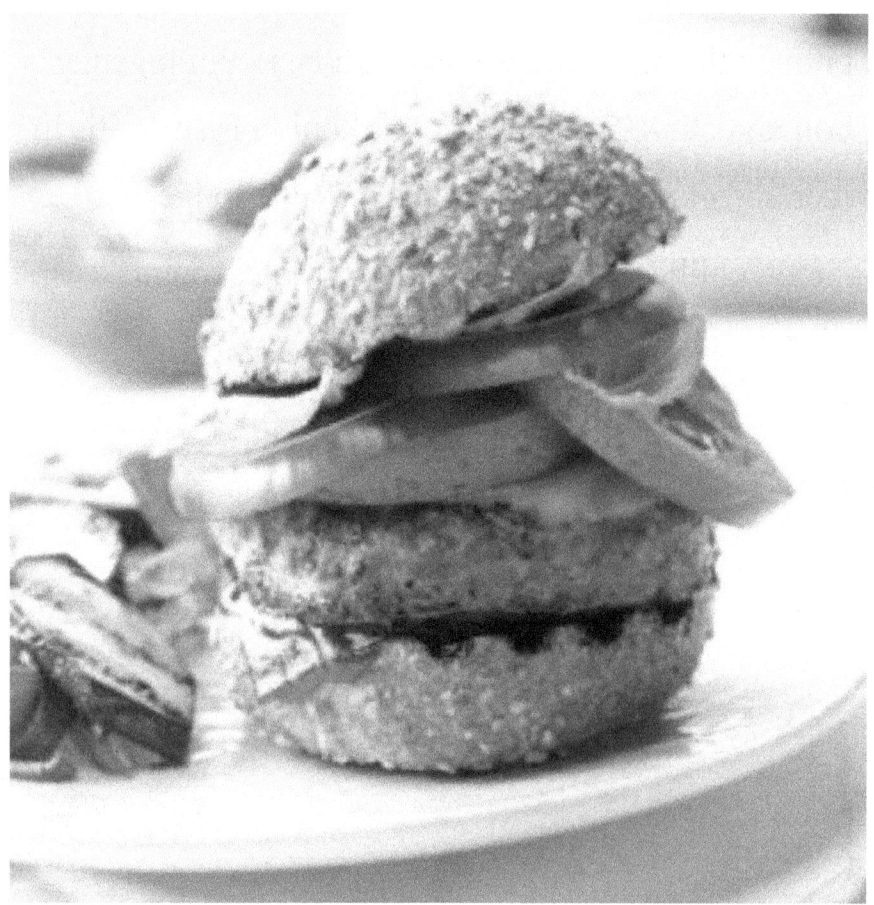

Prep Time: 15mins

Cook Time: 15mins

Total Time: 30 mins

Servings: 4

Ingredients

- ☐ 1/4 cup chopped fresh basil
- ☐ 3 tablespoons mesquite smoke-flavoured barbecue sauce
- ☐ 2 tablespoons quick-cooking oats or oat bran
- ☐ 1 garlic clove, minced
- ☐ 1/4 teaspoon garlic salt
- ☐ 1/8 teaspoon pepper
- ☐ 1 pound lean ground turkey
- ☐ 4 whole wheat or multigrain hamburger buns, split
- ☐ Optional toppings: sliced provolone cheese, red onion slices, sliced tomato, fresh basil leaves and additional barbecue sauce

Directions

1. In a bowl that is large combine basil, barbecue sauce, oats, garlic, garlic salt and pepper. Add turkey; mix lightly but thoroughly. Shape into four 1/2-in.-thick patties.

2. On a grill that is lightly greased, grill burgers, covered, over medium heat 5-7 minutes for each side or until a thermometer reads 165°. Let the grill buns over medium heat then cut side down, for 30-60 seconds or until toasted. Serve burgers on buns with toppings that you choose

4. Fruit & Almond Bites

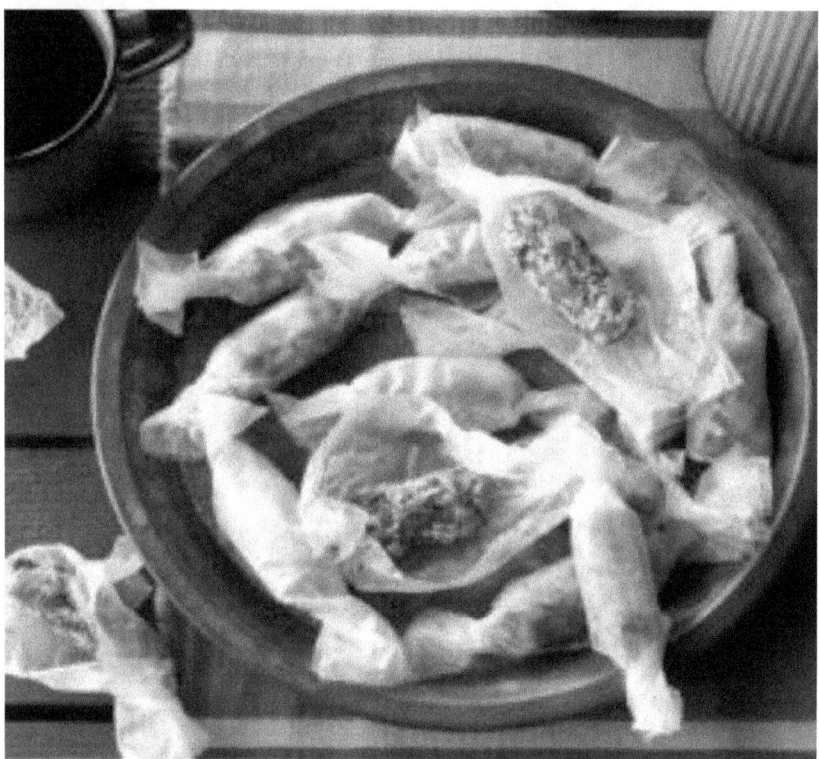

Prep Time: 10 mins

Cook Time: 20 mins

Total Time: 30 mins

Servings: 6

Ingredients

- [ ] 3-3/4 cups sliced almonds, divided
- [ ] 1/4 teaspoon almond extract
- [ ] 1/4 cup honey
- [ ] 2 cups finely chopped dried apricots
- [ ] 1 cup finely chopped dried cherries or cranberries
- [ ] 1 cup finely chopped pistachios, toasted

Directions

1. Place 1-1/4 cups almonds in a food processor; pulse until finely chopped. Remove almonds to a smaller bowl; keep for coating.

2. Add remaining 2-1/2 cups almonds to food processor; pulse until finely chopped. Add extract. While processing, add honey gradually. Remove to a bowl that is large stir in apricots and cherries. Separate the mixture into 6parts; keep in shape each into a 1/2-in.-thick roll. Wrap in plastic; refrigerate until firm, about 60 minutes.

3. Unwrap and cut rolls into 1-1/2-in. pieces. Roll 1 / 2 of the pieces in reserved almonds, pressing gently to adhere. Roll half that is remaining pistachios. If desired, wrap individually in waxed paper, twisting ends to shut. Store in airtight containers, layered between waxed paper if unwrapped.

5. Turkey Medallions with Tomato Salad

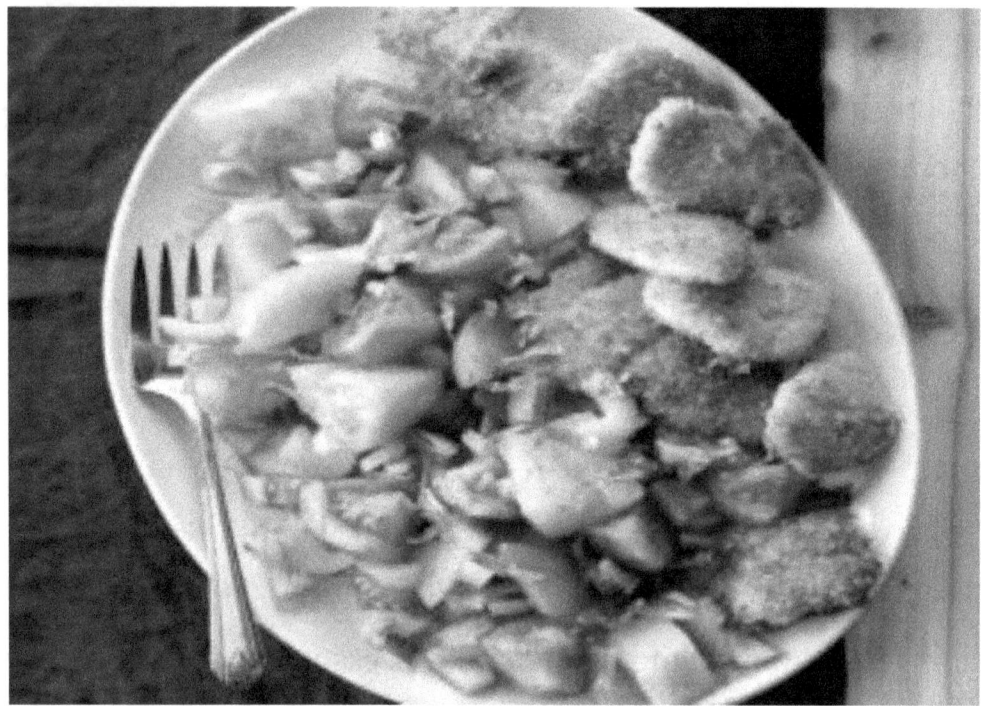

Prep Time: 30 mins
Cook Time: 15 mins
Total Time: 45 mins
Servings: 6

Ingredients

- [ ] 2 tablespoons olive oil
- [ ] 1 tablespoon red wine vinegar
- [ ] 1/2 teaspoon sugar
- [ ] 1/4 teaspoon dried oregano
- [ ] 1/4 teaspoon salt
- [ ] 1 medium green pepper, coarsely chopped
- [ ] 1 celery rib, coarsely chopped
- [ ] 1/4 cup chopped red onion
- [ ] 1 tablespoon thinly sliced fresh basil
- [ ] 3 medium tomatoes

Turkey:

- [ ] 1 large egg
- [ ] 2 tablespoons lemon juice
- [ ] 1 cup panko (Japanese) bread crumbs
- [ ] 1/2 cup grated Parmesan cheese
- [ ] 1/2 cup finely chopped walnuts
- [ ] 1 teaspoon lemon-pepper seasoning
- [ ] 1 package (20 ounces) turkey breast tenderloins
- [ ] 1/4 teaspoon salt
- [ ] 1/4 teaspoon pepper
- [ ] 3 tablespoons olive oil
- [ ] Additional fresh basil

Directions

1. Whisk together first five ingredients. Stir in green pepper, celery, onion and basil. Cut tomatoes into wedges; cut wedges in half. Stir into pepper mixture.

2. With a small bowl, stir together egg and lemon juice. In another shallow skillet, toss breadcrumbs with cheese, walnuts and lemon pepper.

3. Cut tenderloins crosswise into 1-in. slices; flatten slices with a meat mallet to 1/2-in. thickness. Sprinkle with salt and pepper. Dip in egg mixture, then in crumb mixture, patting to adhere.

4. In a large skillet, heat 1 tablespoon oil over medium-high heat. Put together the third to turkey; cook until golden brown, 2-3 minutes per side. Repeat twice with remaining oil and turkey. Serve with tomato join together.

6. Strawberry-Blue Cheese Steak Salad

Prep Time: 15 mins
Cook Time: 15 mins
Total Time: 30 mins
Servings: 4

Ingredients

- ☐ 1 beef top sirloin steak (3/4 inch thick and 1 pound)
- ☐ 1/2 teaspoon salt
- ☐ 1/4 teaspoon pepper
- ☐ 2 teaspoons olive oil
- ☐ 2 tablespoons lime juice

Salad:

- ☐ 1 bunch romaine, torn (about 10 cups)
- ☐ 2 cups fresh strawberries, halved
- ☐ 1/4 cup thinly sliced red onion
- ☐ 1/4 cup crumbled blue cheese
- ☐ 1/4 cup chopped walnuts, toasted
- ☐ Reduced-fat balsamic vinaigrette

Directions

1. Season steak with pepper and salt. In a skillet that is large heat oil over medium heat. Put up steak; cook 5-7 minutes for each part side until meat arrived desired doneness (for medium-rare, a thermometer should read 135°; medium, 140°; medium-well, 145°). Remove from pan; let stand five minutes. Shape the steak into bite-size strips together with lime juice.

2. On a platter, combine romaine, strawberries and onion; top with steak. Sprinkle with cheese and walnuts. Serve with vinaigrette.

7. Skinny Quinoa Veggie Dip

Prep Time: 20 mins

Cook Time: 15 mins

Total Time: 35 mins

Servings: 32

Ingredients

- ☐ 2 cans (15 ounces) black beans, rinsed and drained
- ☐ 1-1/2 teaspoons ground cumin
- ☐ 1-1/2 teaspoons paprika
- ☐ 1/2 teaspoon cayenne pepper
- ☐ 1-2/3 cups water, divided
- ☐ Salt and pepper to taste
- ☐ 2/3 cup quinoa, rinsed
- ☐ 5 tablespoons lime juice, divided
- ☐ 2 medium ripe avocados, peeled and coarsely chopped
- ☐ 2 tablespoons plus 3/4 cup sour cream, divided
- ☐ 1/4 cup minced fresh cilantro
- ☐ 3 plum tomatoes, chopped
- ☐ 3/4 cup peeled, seeded and finely chopped cucumber
- ☐ 3/4 cup finely chopped zucchini
- ☐ 1/4 cup finely chopped red onion
- ☐ Cucumber slices

Directions

1. Pulse beans, cumin, paprika, and cayenne in a 1/3 cup in a food processor until smooth. Add pepper and salt to taste.

2. In a saucepan that is large cook quinoa with remaining 1-1/3 cups water relating to package directions. Fluff with a fork; sprinkle with 2 tablespoons lime juice. Put aside. Meanwhile, mash together avocados, 2 tablespoons sour cream, cilantro and remaining juice that is lime.

3. In a 2-1/2-qt. dish, layer bean mixture, quinoa, avocado mixture, remaining cream that is sour tomatoes, chopped cucumber, zucchini and onion.

8. Roasted Sweet Potato & Chickpea Pitas

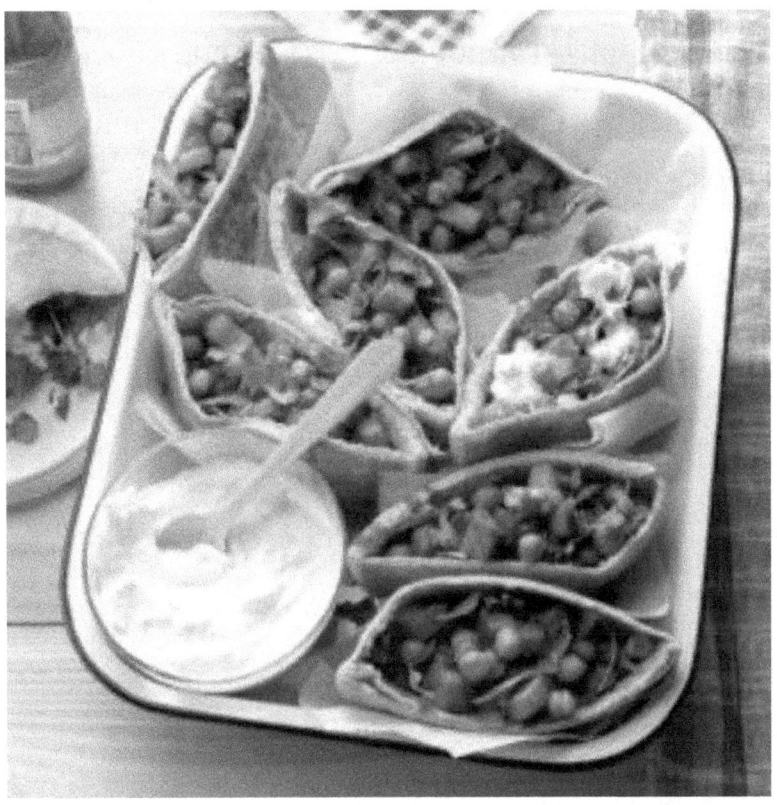

Prep Time: 20 mins

Cook Time: 10 mins

Total Time: 30 mins

Servings : 6

Ingredients

- ☐ 2 medium sweet potatoes (about 1-1/4 pounds), peeled and cubed
- ☐ 2 cans (15 ounces each) chickpeas or garbanzo beans, rinsed and drained
- ☐ 1 medium red onion, chopped
- ☐ 3 tablespoons canola oil, divided
- ☐ 2 teaspoons garam masala
- ☐ 1/2 teaspoon salt, divided
- ☐ 2 garlic cloves, minced
- ☐ 1 cup plain Greek yoghurt
- ☐ 1 tablespoon lemon juice
- ☐ 1 teaspoon ground cumin
- ☐ 2 cups arugula or baby spinach
- ☐ 12 whole-wheat pita pocket halves, warmed
- ☐ 1/4 cup minced fresh cilantro

Directions

1. Preheat oven to 400°. Put the potatoes in a wide microwave-safe skillet; microwave, covered, on high 5 minutes. Turn in chickpeas and onion; toss with 2 tsp oil, garam masala and 1/4 teaspoon salt.

2. Spread into a 15x10x1-in. pan. Roast the potatoes until it soft, about 15 minutes. Cool slightly.

3. Place garlic and remaining oil in a small microwave-safe bowl; microwave on high until garlic is lightly browned, 1 to 1-1/2 minutes. Turn in yoghurt, lemon juice, cumin and remaining salt.

4. Toss potato together with arugula. Use spoon to pitas; top with sauce and cilantro.

10. Pretty Peach Tart

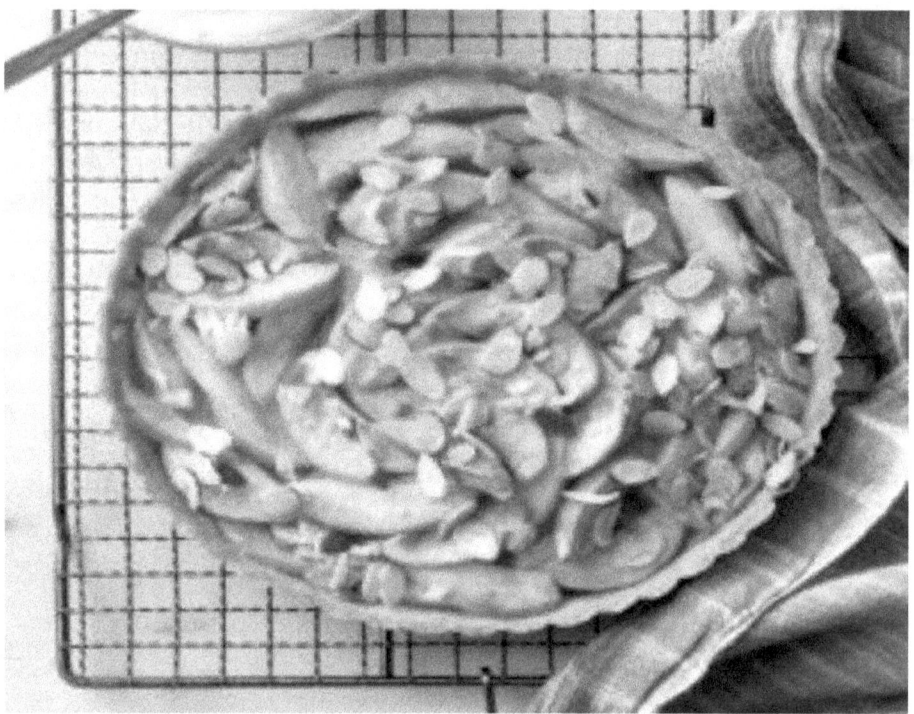

Prep Time: 30 mins

Cook Time: 40 mins

Total Time: 40 mins + cooling

Servings : 8

Ingredients

- ☐ 1/4 cup butter, softened
- ☐ 3 tablespoons sugar
- ☐ 1/4 teaspoon ground nutmeg
- ☐ 1 cup all-purpose flour

Filling:

- ☐ 2 pounds peaches (about 7 medium), sliced and peeled
- ☐ 1/3 cup sugar
- ☐ 2 tablespoons all-purpose flour
- ☐ 1/4 teaspoon ground cinnamon
- ☐ 1/8 teaspoon almond extract
- ☐ 1/4 cup sliced almonds
- ☐ Whipped cream, optional

Directions

1. Preheat oven to 375°. Cream butter, nutmeg and sugar until light and fluffy. Beat in flour until blended (mixture shall be dry). Press firmly onto the bottom or over sides of an ungreased 9-in. a fluted pan that is the tart removable bottom.

2. Place on a baking sheet. Bake on an oven that is middle until lightly browned, 10-12 minutes. Cool on a wire rack.

3. In a bowl that is large toss peaches with sugar, flour, cinnamon and extracts; add to crust. Sprinkle with almonds.

4. Bake tart on a lower life expectancy oven rack until crust is golden brown and peaches are tender 40-45 minutes. Cool on a wire rack. If desired, serve with whipped cream.

11. Simple Asparagus Soup

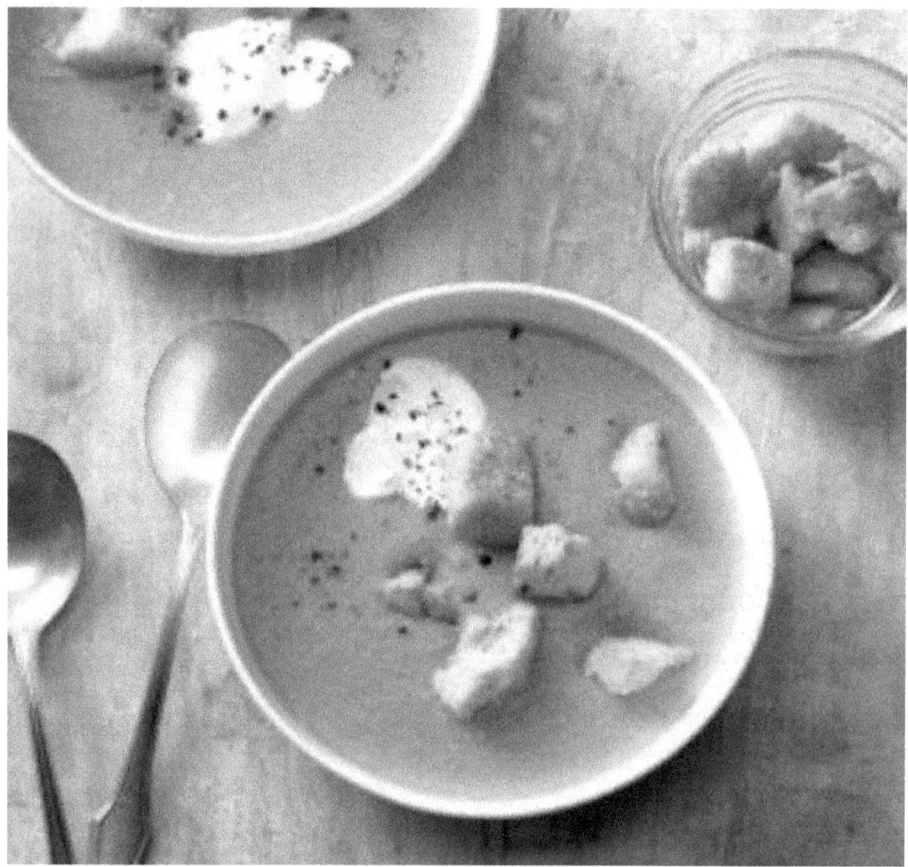

Prep Time: 20 mins

Cook Time: 55 mins

Total Time: 1 hr 15 mins

Servings: 12

Ingredients

- ☐ 1 tablespoon butter
- ☐ 1 tablespoon olive oil
- ☐ 2 pounds fresh asparagus, trimmed and cut into 1-inch pieces
- ☐ 1 medium onion, chopped
- ☐ 1 medium carrot, thinly sliced
- ☐ 1/2 teaspoon salt
- ☐ 1/4 teaspoon pepper
- ☐ 1/4 teaspoon dried thyme
- ☐ 2/3 cup uncooked long-grain brown rice
- ☐ 6 cups reduced-sodium chicken broth
- ☐ Reduced-fat sour cream, optional
- ☐ Salad croutons, optional

Directions

1. In a 6-qt. stockpot, heat butter and oil over medium heat. Stir in vegetables and seasonings; cook until vegctables are tender, 8-10 minutes, stirring occasionally.

2. Stir in rice and broth; bring to a boil. Reduce heat; simmer, covered, until rice is tender, 40-45 minutes, stirring occasionally.

3. Puree soup using an immersion blender, or cool slightly and puree the soup in batches in a blender. Return to pot and heat through. If desired, serve with sour

   cream and croutons.

Freeze option: Freeze cooled soup in freezer containers. To use, partially thaw in refrigerator overnight (soup may separate). In a saucepan, reheat to boiling, whisking until blended.

12. Whole Grain Banana Pancakes

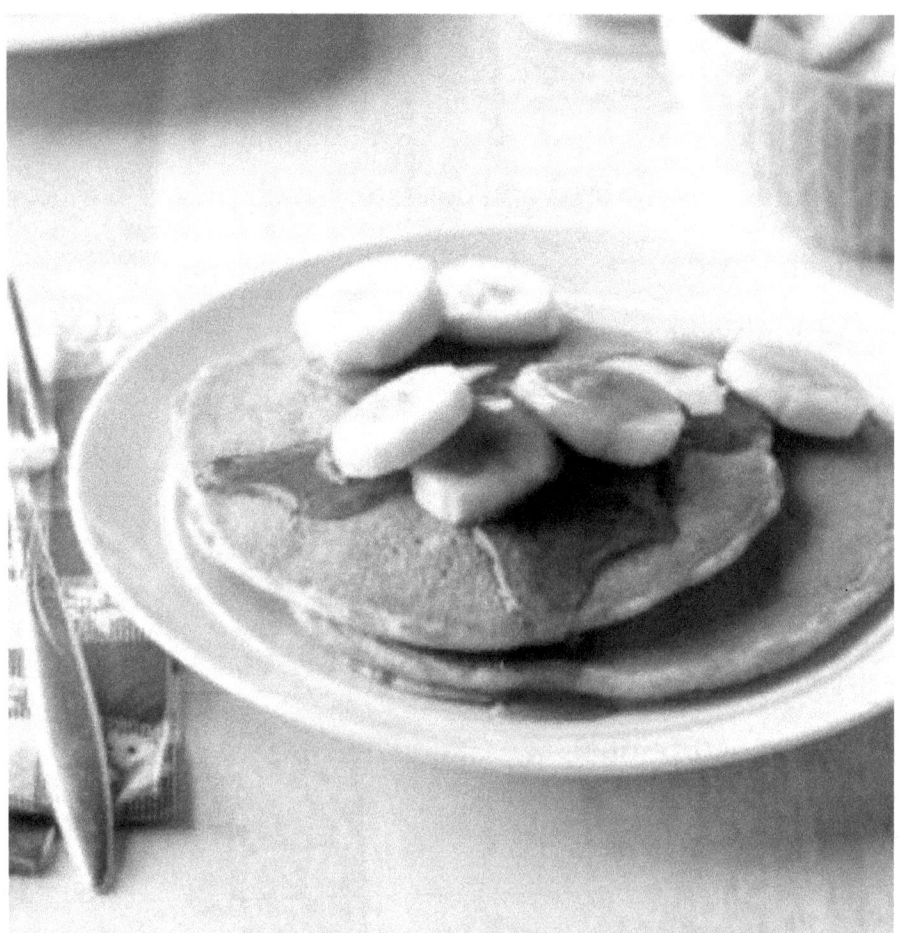

Prep Time: 10 mins

Cook Time: 20 mins

Total Time: 30 min.

Servings: 8

Ingredients

- ☐ 1 cup whole wheat flour
- ☐ 1 cup all-purpose flour
- ☐ 4 teaspoons baking powder
- ☐ 1 teaspoon ground cinnamon
- ☐ 1/2 teaspoon salt
- ☐ 2 large eggs
- ☐ 2 cups fat-free milk
- ☐ 2/3 cup mashed ripe banana (about 1 medium)
- ☐ 1 tablespoon olive oil
- ☐ 1 tablespoon maple syrup
- ☐ 1/2 teaspoon vanilla extract
- ☐ Sliced bananas and additional syrup, optional

Directions

1. Whisk together first 5 ingredients. In another bowl, whisk together eggs, milk, mashed banana, oil, 1 tablespoon syrup and vanilla. Add to flour mixture; stir just until moistened.

2. Preheat a griddle coated with cooking spray over medium heat. Pour batter by 1/4 cup each onto griddle; cook until bubbles on top begin to pop and bottoms are golden brown. Turn; cook until the second side is golden brown. If desired, serve with sliced bananas and additional syrup.

Freeze option: Freeze cooled pancakes between layers of waxed paper in a freezer container or plastic freezer bag. To use, place pancakes on an ungreased baking sheet, cover with foil and reheat in a preheated 375° oven until heated through 10-15 minutes. Or, place a stack of 2pancakes on a microwave-safe plate and microwave on high until heated through, 45-60 seconds.

13. Almond-Chai Granola

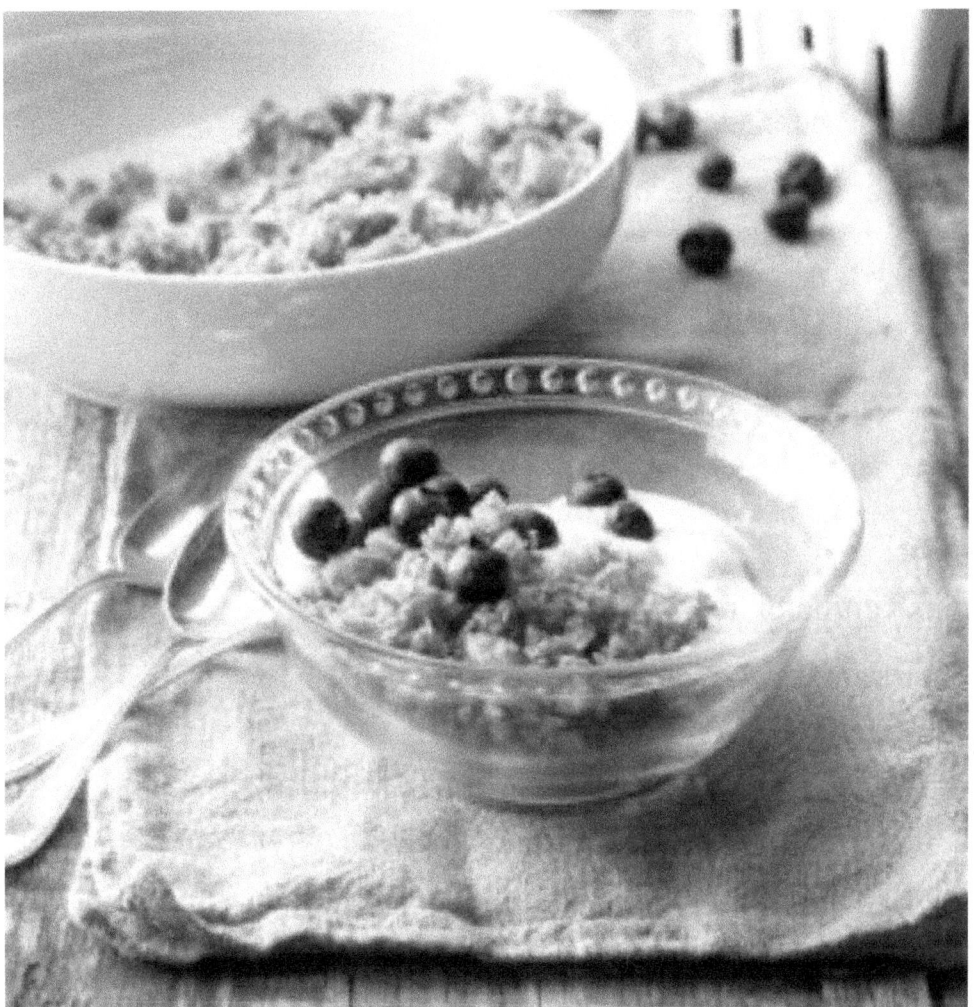

Prep Time: 20 mins

Cook Time: 1hr 15 mins

Total Time: 1 hr 30 mins

Servings: 8

Ingredients

- [ ] 2 chai tea bags
- [ ] 1/4 cup boiling water
- [ ] 3 cups quick-cooking oats
- [ ] 2 cups almonds, coarsely chopped
- [ ] 1 cup sweetened shredded coconut
- [ ] 1/2 cup honey
- [ ] 1/4 cup olive oil
- [ ] 1/3 cup sugar
- [ ] 2 teaspoons vanilla extract
- [ ] 3/4 teaspoon salt
- [ ] 3/4 teaspoon ground cinnamon
- [ ] 3/4 teaspoon ground nutmeg
- [ ] 1/4 teaspoon ground cardamom

Directions

1. Preheat oven to 250°. Steep tea bags in boiling water five full minutes. Meanwhile, combine oats, almonds and coconut. Discard tea bags; stir ingredients that are remaining tea. Pour tea mixture over oat mixture; mix well to coat.

2. Spread evenly in a greased 15x10-in. rimmed pan. Bake until golden brown, stirring every 20 minutes, about 1-1/4 hours. Cool thoroughly without stirring; store in an airtight container.

14. Black Bean & Sweet Potato Rice Bowls

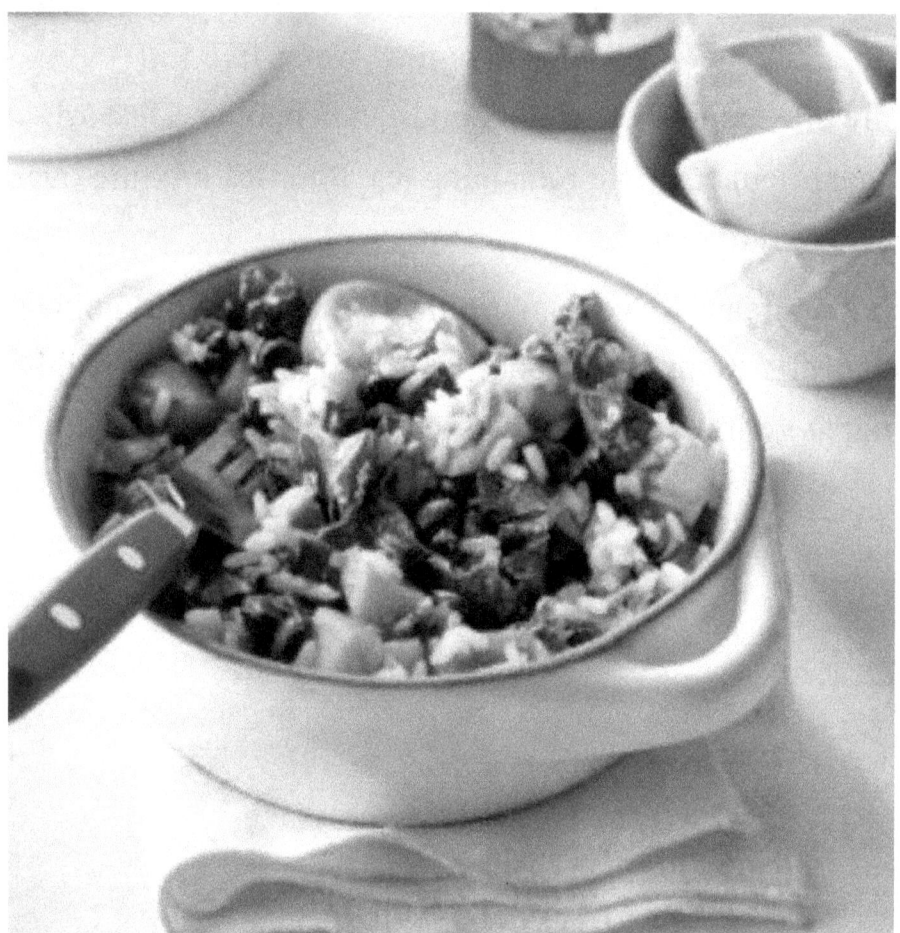

Prep Time: 5 mins

Cook Time: 25 mins

Total Time: 30 min.

Servings : 4

Ingredients

- ☐ 3/4 cup uncooked long-grain rice
- ☐ 1/4 teaspoon garlic salt
- ☐ 1-1/2 cups water
- ☐ 3 tablespoons olive oil, divided
- ☐ 1 large sweet potato, peeled and diced
- ☐ 1 medium red onion, finely chopped
- ☐ 4 cups chopped fresh kale (tough stems removed)
- ☐ 1 can (15 ounces) black beans, rinsed and drained
- ☐ 2 tablespoons sweet chilli sauce
- ☐ Lime wedges, optional
- ☐ Additional sweet chilli sauce, optional

Directions

1. Place rice, garlic salt and water in a saucepan that is large bring to a boil. Reduce heat; simmer, covered until water is absorbed and rice is tender minutes that are 15-20. Separate it from heat; let cool for five minutes.

2. Meanwhile, in a skillet that is large heat 2 tablespoons oil over medium-high heat; sauté sweet potato 8 minutes. Add onion; stir and cook until potato is tender 4-6 minutes. Add kale; stir and cook until tender, 3-5 minutes. Stir in beans; heat through.

3. Gently stir 2 tablespoons chili sauce and oil that is remaining rice; add to potato mixture. If desired, serve with lime wedges and chili that are additional.

15. The Ultimate Fish Tacos

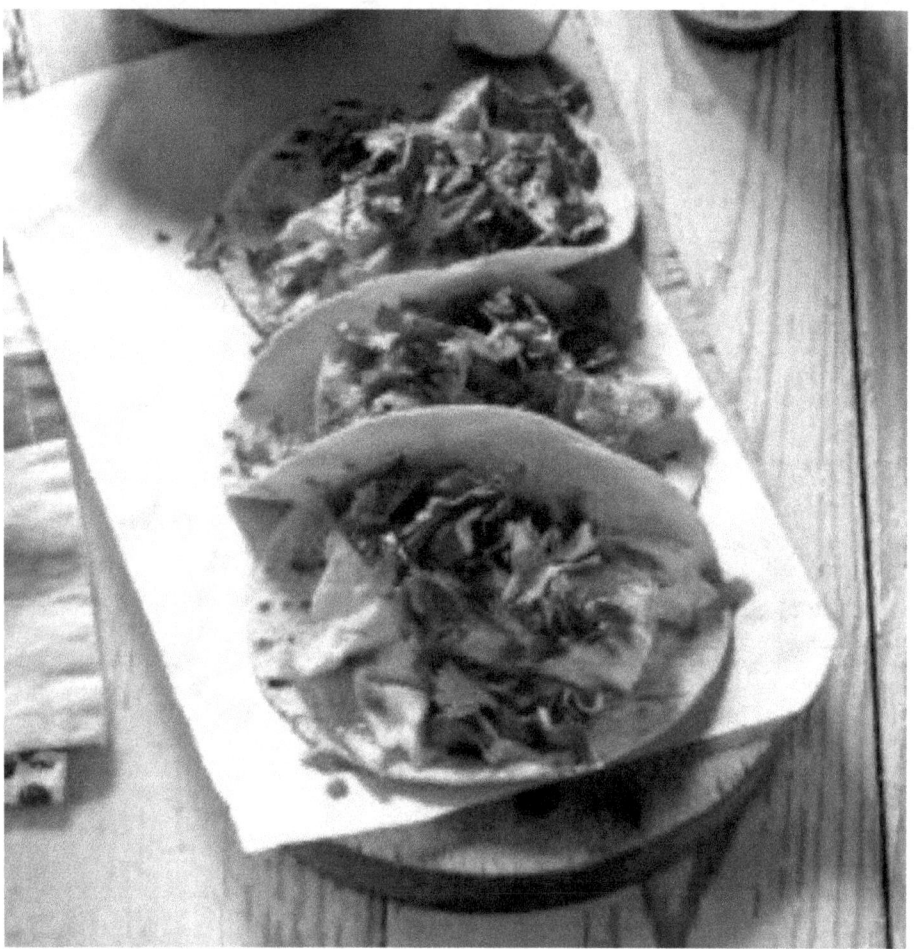

Prep Time: 20 mins
Cook Time: 10 mins
Total Time: 30 mins
Servings: 6

Ingredients

- ☐ 1/4 cup olive oil
- ☐ 1 teaspoon ground cardamom
- ☐ 1 teaspoon paprika
- ☐ 1 teaspoon salt
- ☐ 1 teaspoon pepper
- ☐ 6 mahi-mahi fillets (6 ounces each)
- ☐ 12 corn tortillas (6 inches)
- ☐ 2 cups chopped red cabbage
- ☐ 1 cup chopped fresh cilantro
- ☐ Salsa Verde, optional
- ☐ 2 medium limes, cut into wedges
- ☐ Hot pepper sauce (Tapatio preferred)

Directions

1. In a 13x9-in. baking dish, whisk the initial 5 ingredients. Add fillets; look to the coat. Refrigerate, covered, thirty minutes.

2. Drain discard and fish marinade. On a grill that is oiled, grill mahi-mahi, covered, over medium-high heat (or broil 4 in. from heat) until it flakes easily with a fork, 4-5 minutes per side. Remove fish. Put in the tortillas on grill rack; heat 30-45 seconds. Keep warm.

3. To put together, divide fish among the list of tortillas; layer with red cabbage, cilantro and, if desired, Salsa Verde. Squeeze a lime that is little and hot pepper sauce over fish mixture; fold sides of tortilla throughout the mixture. Serve with lime wedges and pepper sauce that is additional.

16. Chickpea Mint Tabbouleh

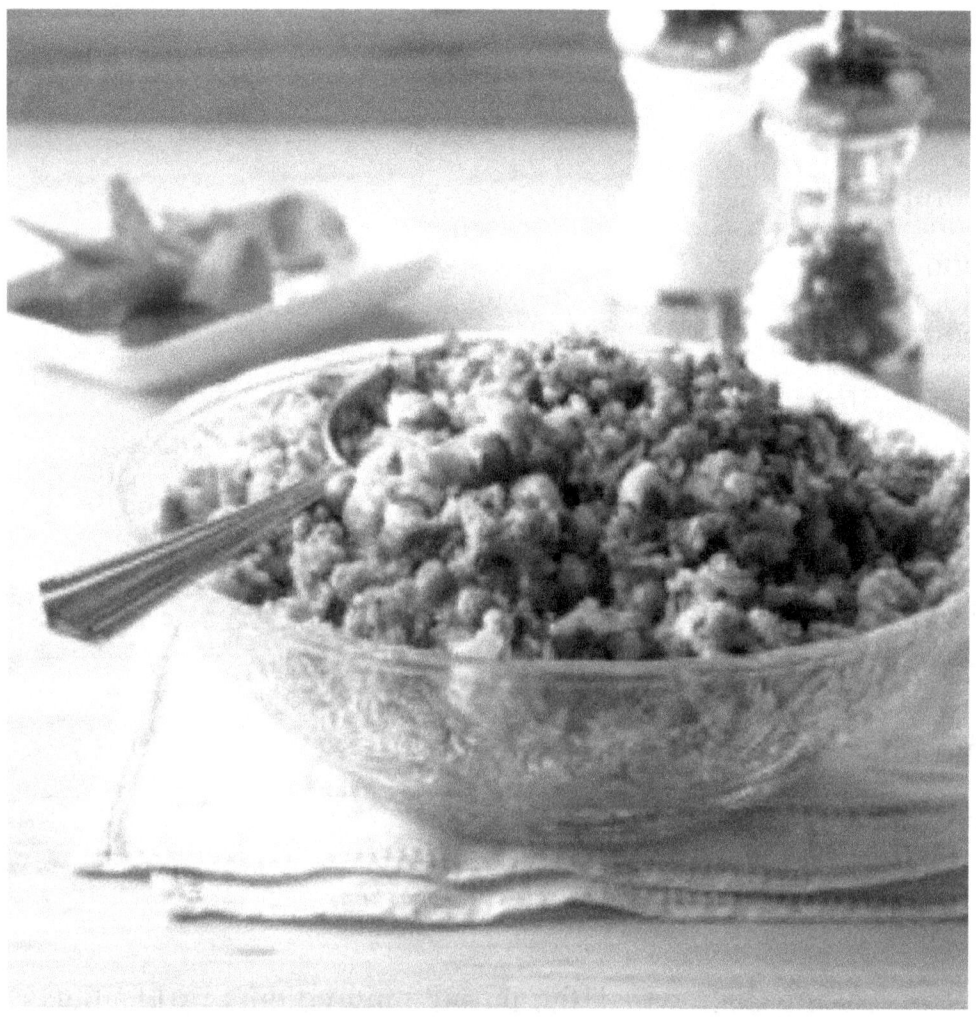

Prep Time: 15 mins

Cook Time: 15 mins

Total Time: 30 mins

Servings: 4

Ingredients

- [ ] 1 cup bulgur
- [ ] 2 cups of water
- [ ] 1 cup fresh or frozen peas (about 5 ounces), thawed
- [ ] 1 can (15 ounces) chickpeas or garbanzo beans, rinsed and drained
- [ ] 1/2 cup minced fresh parsley
- [ ] 1/4 cup minced fresh mint
- [ ] 1/4 cup olive oil
- [ ] 2 tablespoons julienned soft sun-dried tomatoes (not packed in oil)
- [ ] 2 tablespoons lemon juice
- [ ] 1/2 teaspoon salt
- [ ] 1/4 teaspoon pepper

Directions

1. In a saucepan that is large combine bulgur and water; bring to a boil. Reduce heat; simmer, covered, ten full minutes. Stir in fresh or peas that are frozen cook, covered, until bulgur and peas are tender, about five full minutes.

2. Transfer to a bowl that is large. Stir in remaining ingredients. Serve should be made warm, or refrigerate and serve chilled.

17. Sesame Chicken Veggie Wraps

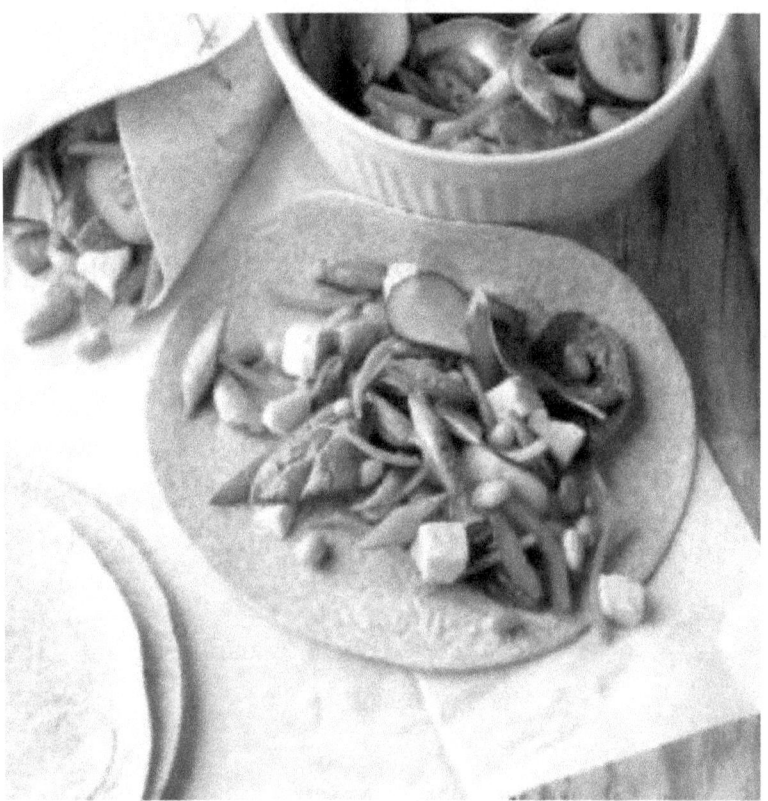

Prep: 10 mins

Cook Time: 20 mins

Total Time: 30 min.

Servings : 8

Ingredients

- ☐ 1 cup frozen shelled edamame

Dressing:

- ☐ 2 tablespoons orange juice
- ☐ 2 tablespoons olive oil
- ☐ 1 teaspoon sesame oil
- ☐ 1/2 teaspoon ground ginger
- ☐ 1/4 teaspoon salt
- ☐ 1/8 teaspoon pepper

Wraps:

- ☐ 2 cups fresh baby spinach
- ☐ 1 cup thinly sliced cucumber
- ☐ 1 cup fresh sugar snap peas, chopped
- ☐ 1/2 cup shredded carrots
- ☐ 1/2 cup thinly sliced sweet red pepper
- ☐ 1 cup chopped cooked chicken breast
- ☐ 8 whole-wheat tortillas (8 inches), room temperature

Directions

1. Cook edamame relating to package directions. Drain; rinse with chilled water and drain well. Whisk ingredients that are together dressing.

In a bowl that is large combine remaining vegetables, chicken and edamame; toss with dressing. Place about 1/2 cup mixture for each tortilla. Fold down part of tortilla and sides of tortilla over filling and roll-up.

18. Ricotta, Tomato & Corn Pasta

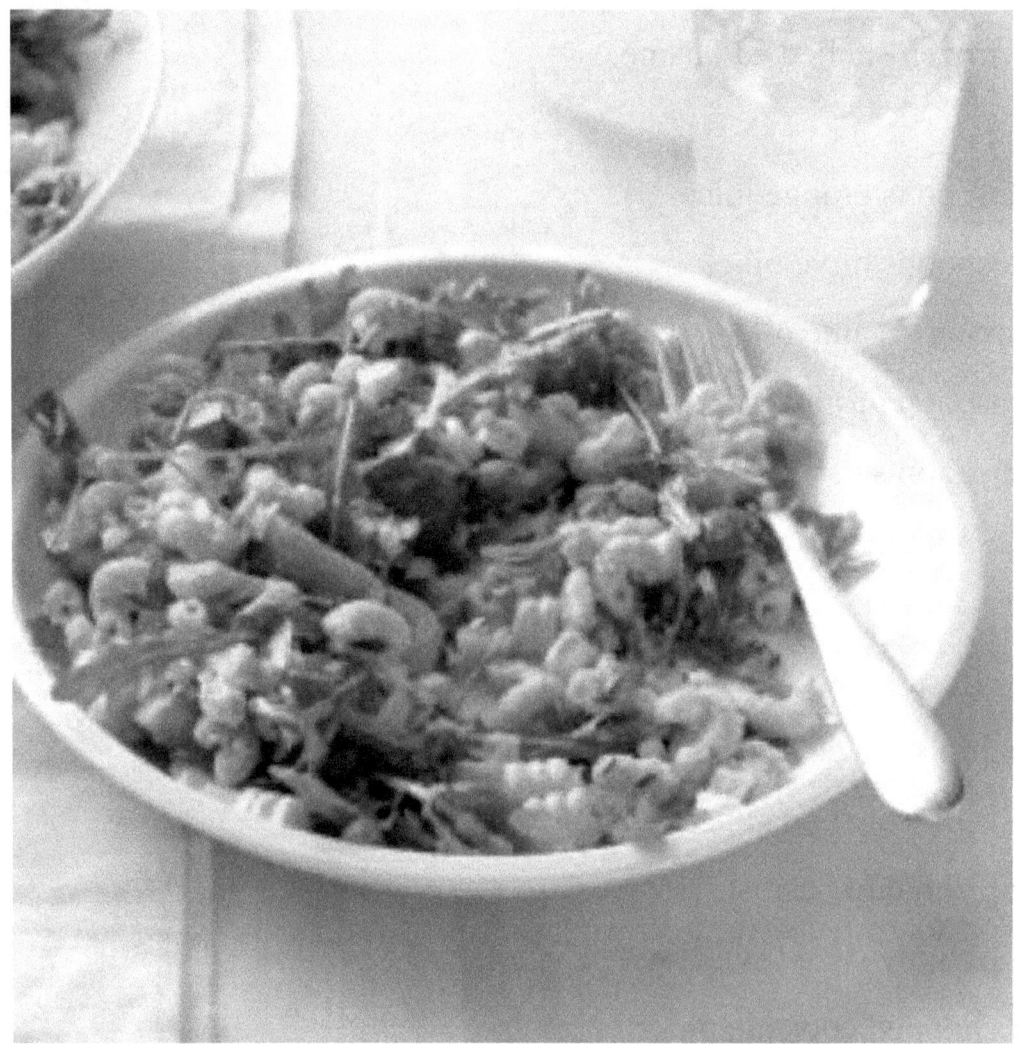

Prep Time: 10 mins

Cook Time: 20 mins

Total Time: 30 mins

Servings: 8

Ingredients

- [ ] 3 cups uncooked whole-wheat elbow macaroni (about 12 ounces)
- [ ] 1 can (15 ounces) cannellini beans, rinsed and drained
- [ ] 2 cups cherry tomatoes, halved
- [ ] 1 cup fresh or frozen corn, thawed
- [ ] 1/2 cup finely chopped red onion
- [ ] 1/2 cup part-skim ricotta cheese
- [ ] 1/4 cup grated Parmesan cheese
- [ ] 2 tablespoons minced fresh basil or 2 teaspoons dried basil
- [ ] 1 tablespoon olive oil
- [ ] 3 garlic cloves, minced
- [ ] 1 teaspoon salt
- [ ] 1 teaspoon minced fresh rosemary or 1/2 teaspoon dried rosemary, crushed
- [ ] 1/2 teaspoon pepper
- [ ] 3 cups arugula or baby spinach
- [ ] Chopped fresh parsley, optional

Directions

1. Cook pasta relating to package directions. Rinse and drain with chilled water; drain well.

2. In a bowl that is large combine beans, tomatoes, corn, onion, ricotta and Parmesan cheeses, basil, oil, garlic, salt, rosemary and pepper. Stir in pasta. Add arugula; toss gently to mix. If desired, sprinkle with parsley. Serve immediately.

19. Pesto Corn Salad with Shrimp

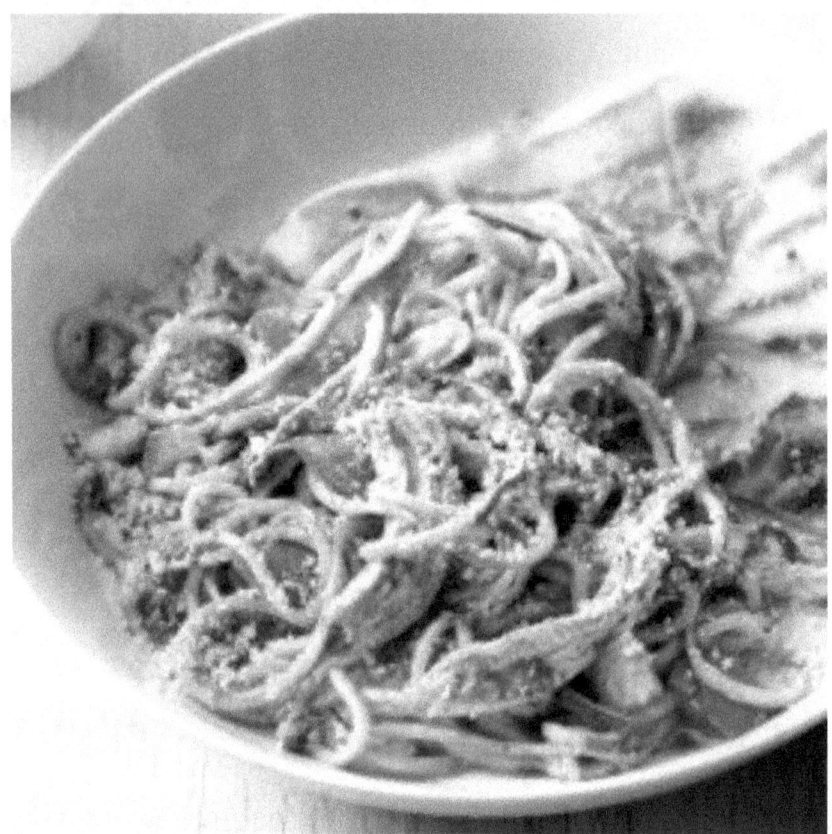

Prep Time: 15 mins

Cook Time: 15 mins

Total Time: 30 min.

Servings : 4

Ingredients

- ☐ 4 medium ears sweet corn, husked
- ☐ 1/2 cup packed fresh basil leaves
- ☐ 1/4 cup olive oil
- ☐ 1/2 teaspoon salt, divided
- ☐ 1-1/2 cups cherry tomatoes halved
- ☐ 1/8 teaspoon pepper
- ☐ 1 medium ripe avocado, peeled and chopped
- ☐ 1 pound uncooked shrimp (31-40 per pound), peeled and deveined

Directions

1. In a pot of boiling water, cook corn until tender, about five full minutes. Drain; cool slightly. Before that, in a food processor, hold basil, oil and 1/4 teaspoon salt until well mixed.

2. Cut corn from place and cob in a bowl. Stir in tomatoes, pepper and salt that is remaining. Add avocado and 2 tablespoons basil mixture; toss gently to mix.

3. Thread shrimp onto metal or soaked wooden skewers; brush with the remaining mixture that is basil. Cover the grill, over medium heat till shrimp turn pink, 2-4 minutes per side. Put away shrimp from skewers; goes well with corn mixture.

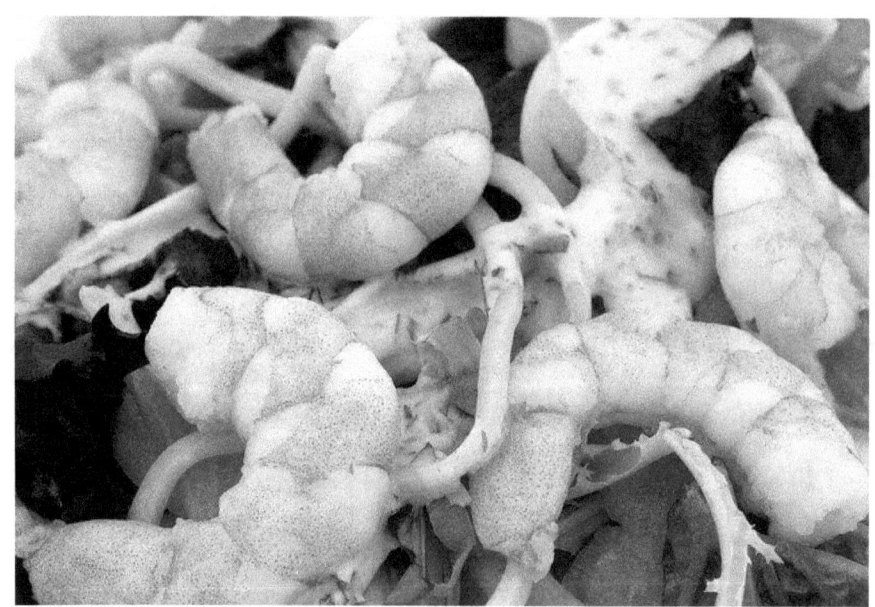

20. Breakfast Sweet Potatoes

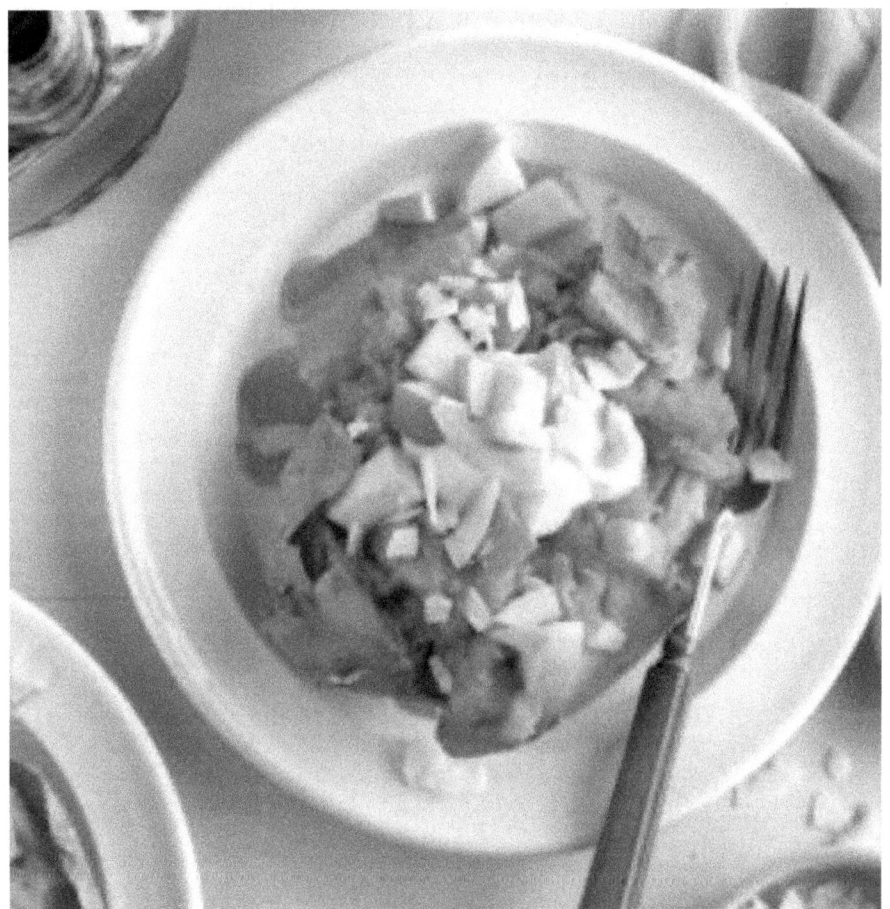

Prep Time: 10 min.

Cook Time: 45 mins

Total Time: 55 min

Servings: 4

Ingredients

- ☐ 4 medium sweet potatoes (about 8 ounces each)
- ☐ 1/2 cup fat-free coconut Greek yoghurt
- ☐ 1 medium apple, chopped
- ☐ 2 tablespoons maple syrup
- ☐ 1/4 cup toasted unsweetened coconut flakes

Directions

1. Preheat oven to 400°. Place potatoes on a baking sheet that is foil-lined. Bake until tender, 45-60 minutes.
2. With a knife that is sharp cut an "X" in each potato. Fluff pulp with a fork. Top with remaining ingredients.

21. Salmon with Horseradish Pistachio Crust

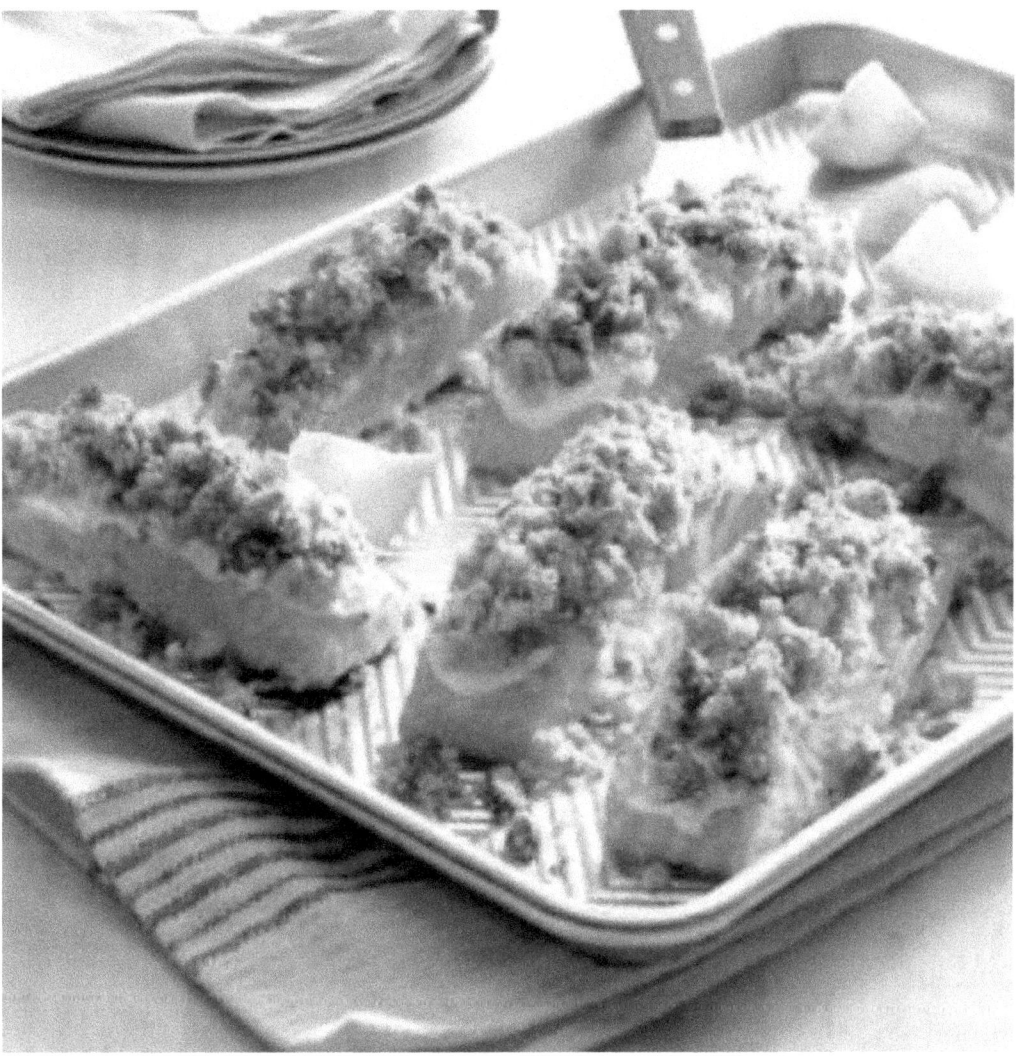

Prep Time: 15 mins
Cook Time:15mins
Total Time: 30 min.
Servings: 6

Ingredients

- ☐ 6 salmon fillets (4 ounces each)
- ☐ 1/3 cup sour cream
- ☐ 2/3 cup dry bread crumbs
- ☐ 2/3 cup chopped pistachios
- ☐ 1/2 cup minced shallots
- ☐ 2 tablespoons olive oil
- ☐ 1 to 2 tablespoons prepared horseradish
- ☐ 1 tablespoon snipped fresh dill or 1 teaspoon dill weed
- ☐ 1/2 teaspoon grated lemon or orange zest
- ☐ 1/4 teaspoon crushed red pepper flakes
- ☐ 1 garlic clove, minced

Directions

1. Preheat oven to 350°. Place salmon, skin side down, in an ungreased 15x10x1-in. baking pan. Spread cream that is sour each fillet. Combine ingredients that are remaining. Pat crumb-nut mixture onto tops of salmon fillets, pressing to assist coating in adhering. Bake until fish just starts to flake easily with a fork, 12-15 minutes.

22. Southwest Shredded Pork Salad

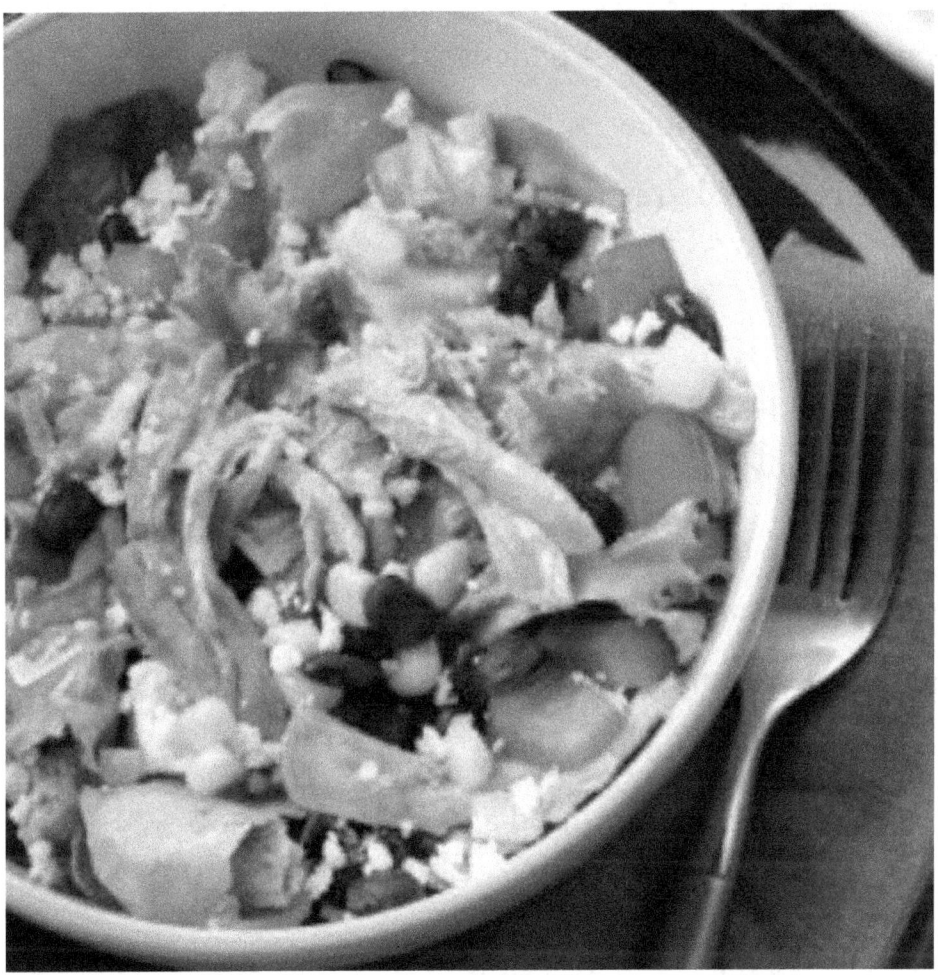

Prep Time: 20 mins

Cook Time: 6 hrs

Total Time: 6 hrs 20 mins

Servings: 12

Ingredients

- [ ] 1 boneless pork loin roast (3 to 4 pounds)
- [ ] 1-1/2 cups apple cider or juice
- [ ] 1 can (4 ounces) chopped green chiles, drained
- [ ] 3 garlic cloves, minced
- [ ] 1-1/2 teaspoons salt
- [ ] 1-1/2 teaspoons hot pepper sauce
- [ ] 1 teaspoon chilli powder
- [ ] 1 teaspoon pepper
- [ ] 1/2 teaspoon ground cumin
- [ ] 1/2 teaspoon dried oregano
- [ ] 12 cups torn mixed salad greens
- [ ] 1 can (15 ounces) black beans, rinsed and drained
- [ ] 2 medium tomatoes, chopped
- [ ] 1 small red onion, chopped
- [ ] 1 cup fresh or frozen corn
- [ ] 1 cup crumbled Cotija or shredded part-skim mozzarella cheese
- [ ] Salad dressing of your choice

Directions

1. Place pork in a 5- or 6-qt. slow cooker. In a small bowl, mix cider, green chiles, garlic, salt, pepper sauce, chilli powder, pepper, cumin and oregano; pour over pork. Cover and cook it on low up to 6-8 hours or until meat is soft.

2. Remove roast from slow cooker; discard cooking juices. Shred pork with 2 forks. Put in the green salad on a large serving platter. Together with pork, black beans, tomatoes, onion, corn and cheese. Serve with salad dressing.

23. White Wine Garlic Chicken

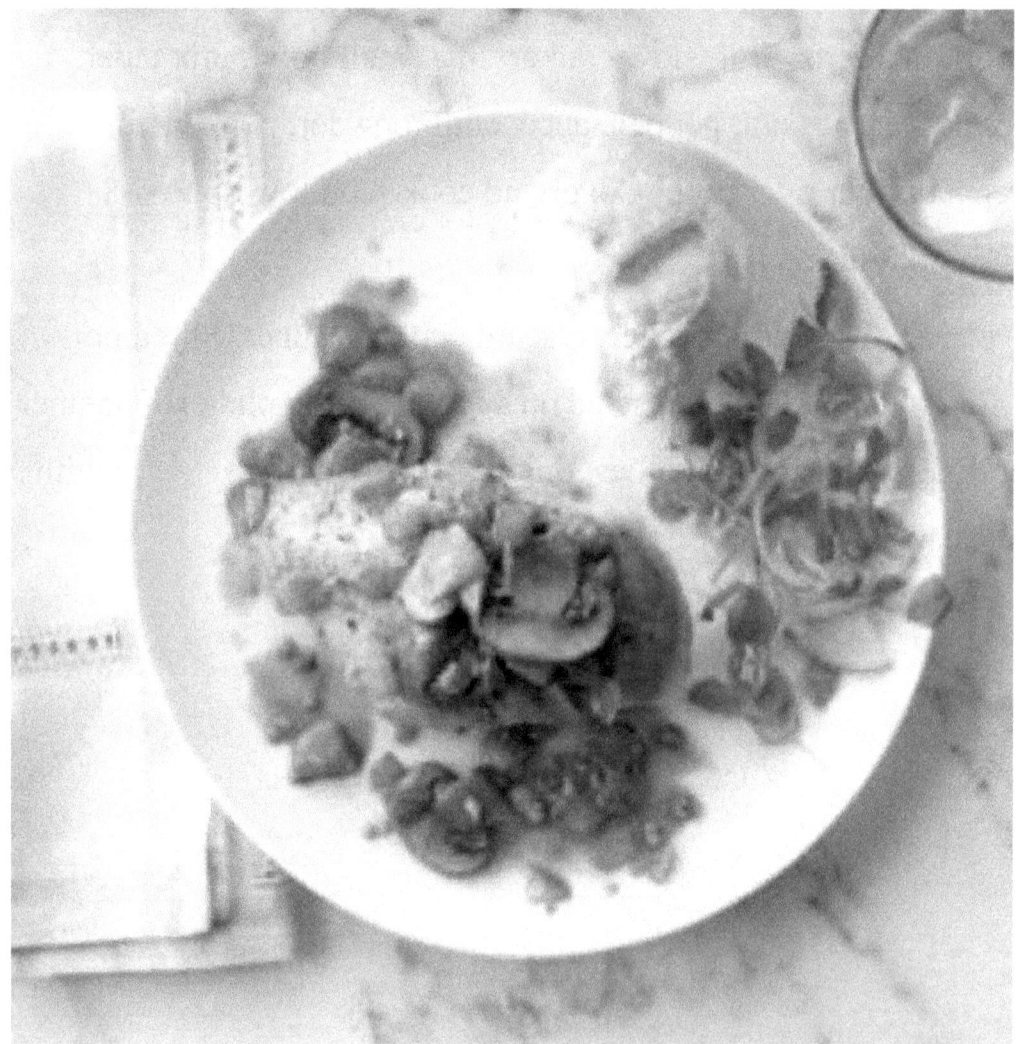

Prep Time:10mins

Cook Time: 20 mins

Total Time: 30 mins

Servings : 6

Ingredients

- ☐ 4 boneless skinless chicken breast halves (6 ounces each)
- ☐ 1/2 teaspoon salt
- ☐ 1/4 teaspoon pepper
- ☐ 1 tablespoon olive oil
- ☐ 2 cups sliced baby portobello mushrooms (about 6 ounces)
- ☐ 1 medium onion, chopped
- ☐ 2 garlic cloves, minced
- ☐ 1/2 cup dry white wine or reduced-sodium chicken broth

Directions

1. Pound chicken breasts with a meat mallet to 1/2-in. thickness; sprinkle with salt and pepper. In a large skillet, heat oil over medium heat; cook chicken until no longer pink, 5-6 minutes per side. Remove from pan; keep warm.

2. Add mushrooms and onion to pan; cook and stir over medium-high heat until tender and lightly browned, 2-3 minutes. Add garlic; cook and stir 30 seconds. Include wine; add to a boil, stirring to loosen browned bits from iron pan. Cook until water is slightly reduced, 1-2 minutes; serve with chicken.

24. Edamame Salad with Sesame Ginger Dressing

Prep Time: 15 mins

Total Time: 15 min.

Servings: 6

Ingredients

- ☐ 6 cups baby kale salad blend (about 5 ounces)
- ☐ 1 can (15 ounces) garbanzo beans *or* chickpeas, rinsed and drained
- ☐ 2 cups frozen shelled edamame (about 10 ounces), thawed
- ☐ 3 clementines, peeled and segmented
- ☐ 1 cup fresh bean sprouts
- ☐ 1/2 cup salted peanuts
- ☐ 2 green onions, diagonally sliced
- ☐ 1/2 cup sesame ginger salad dressing

Directions

1. Divide salad blend among 6 bowls. Add up with the remaining ingredients except salad dressing. Serve with dressing.

25. Cilantro Lime Shrimp

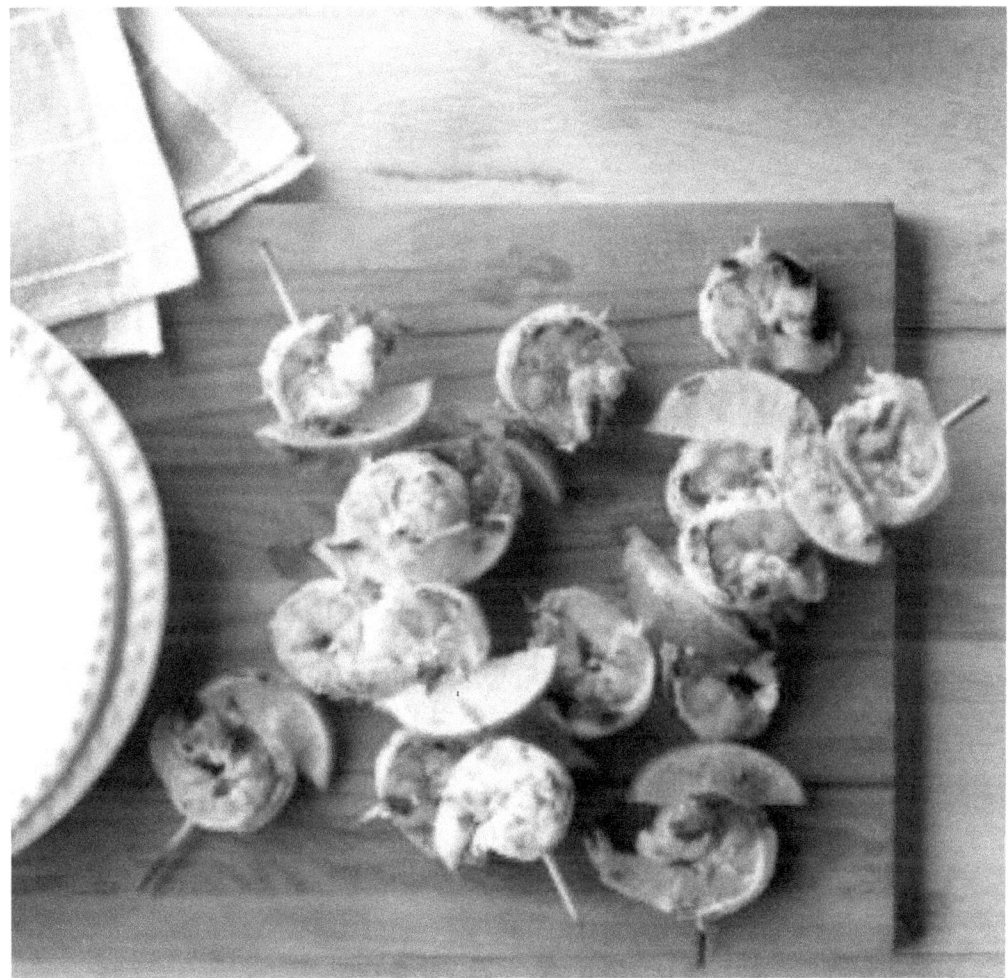

Prep Time: 10 mins

Cook Time: 20 mins

Total Time: 30 min.

Servings: 4

Ingredients

- ☐ 1/3 cup chopped fresh cilantro
- ☐ 1-1/2 teaspoons grated lime zest
- ☐ 1/3 cup lime juice
- ☐ 1 jalapeno pepper, seeded and minced
- ☐ 2 tablespoons olive oil
- ☐ 3 garlic cloves, minced
- ☐ 1/4 teaspoon salt
- ☐ 1/4 teaspoon ground cumin
- ☐ 1/4 teaspoon pepper
- ☐ 1 pound uncooked shrimp (16-20 per pound), peeled and deveined
- ☐ Lime slices

Directions

1. Mix first 9 ingredients; toss with shrimp. Let stand 15 minutes.

2. Thread shrimp and lime slices onto 4 metal or soaked wooden skewers. Cover the grill with medium heat until shrimp turn pink, 2-4 minutes per side.

26. Creamy Lentils with Kale Artichoke Sauté

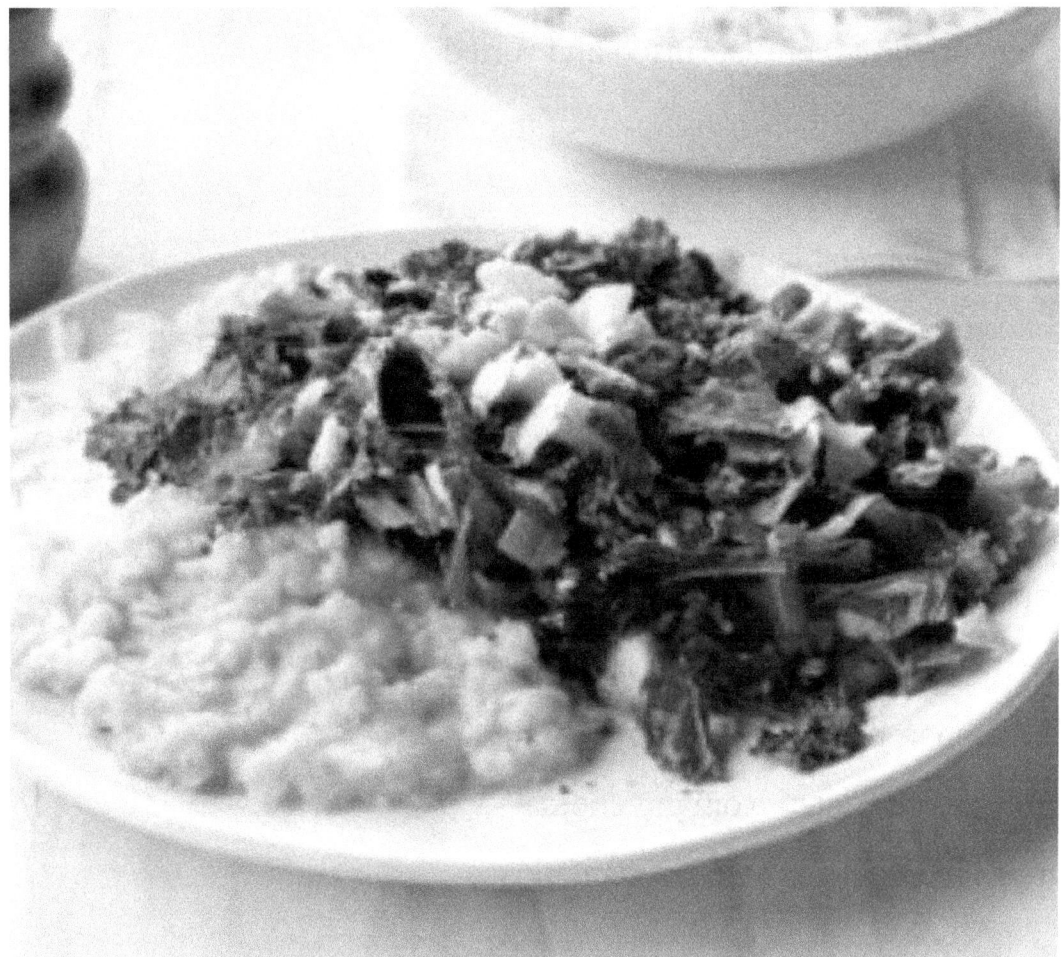

Prep Time: 5 mins
Cook Time: 25 mins
Total Time: 30 mins
Servings : 4

Ingredients

- ☐ 1/2 cup dried red lentils, rinsed and sorted
- ☐ 1/4 teaspoon dried oregano
- ☐ 1/8 teaspoon pepper
- ☐ 1-1/4 cups vegetable broth
- ☐ 1/4 teaspoon sea salt, divided
- ☐ 1 tablespoon olive oil or grapeseed oil
- ☐ 16 cups chopped fresh kale (about 12 ounces)
- ☐ 1 can (14 ounces) water-packed artichoke hearts, drained and chopped
- ☐ 3 garlic cloves, minced
- ☐ 1/2 teaspoon Italian seasoning
- ☐ 2 tablespoons grated Romano cheese
- ☐ 2 cups hot cooked brown or basmati rice

Directions

1. Place first 4 ingredients and 1/8 teaspoon salt in a small saucepan; bring to a boil. Reduce heat; simmer, covered until lentils are tender and liquid is almost absorbed 12-15 minutes. Remove from heat.

2. In a 6-qt. stockpot, heat oil over medium heat. Put little salt, kale and cook, covered, until kale is wilted, 4-5 minutes, stirring occasionally. Again put in artichoke hearts, garlic and Italian seasoning; cook and turn it around every 3 minutes. Separate it from heat; stir in cheese.

3. Serve lentils and kale together over rice.

27. Quinoa Unstuffed Peppers

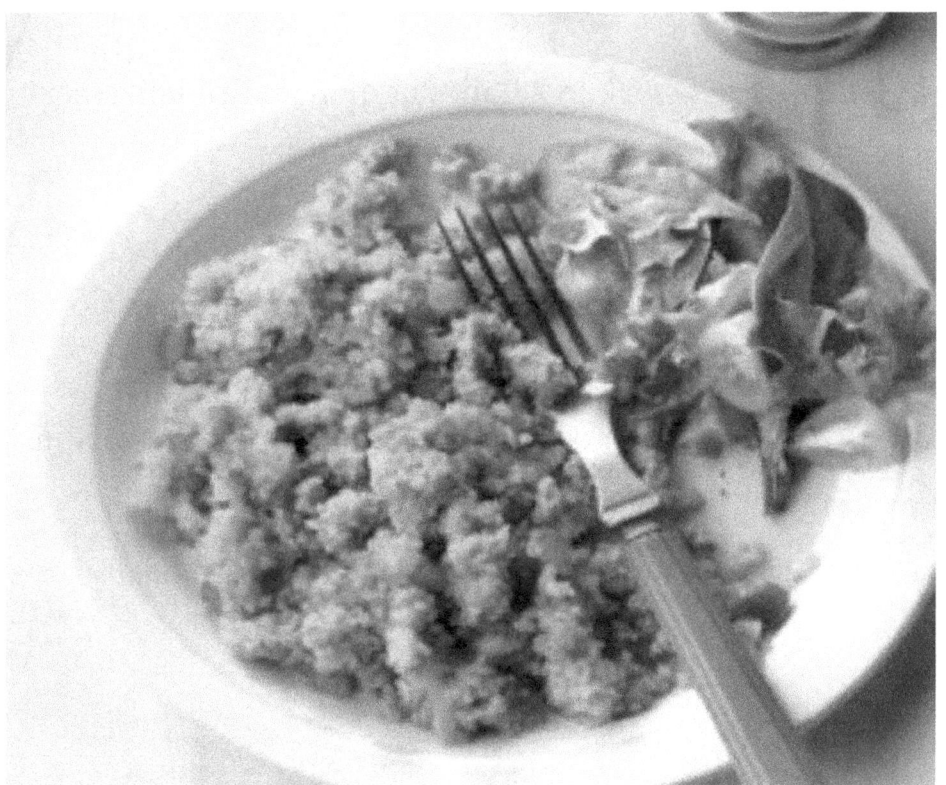

Prep Time: 5 mins
Cook Time: 25 mins
Total Time: 30 min.
Servings : 4

Ingredients

- ☐ 1-1/2 cups vegetable stock
- ☐ 3/4 cup quinoa, rinsed
- ☐ 1 pound Italian turkey sausage links, casings removed
- ☐ 1 medium sweet red pepper, chopped
- ☐ 1 medium green pepper, chopped
- ☐ 3/4 cup chopped sweet onion
- ☐ 1 garlic clove, minced
- ☐ 1/4 teaspoon garam masala
- ☐ 1/4 teaspoon pepper

□   1/8 teaspoon salt

Directions

1. In a small skillet, bring the stock to a boil. Put quinoa. Minimize heat, simmer, and hold until liquid is absorbed, 12-15 minutes. Separate from heat.

2. In a large skillet, cook and crumble sausage with peppers and onion over medium-high heat until no longer pink, 8-10 minutes. Place cooled quinoa mixture in freezer containers. To use, partially thaw in refrigerator overnight. Microwave should be covered, on high in a microwave-safe dish till it is heated through, stirring occasionally.

28. White Beans & Bow Ties

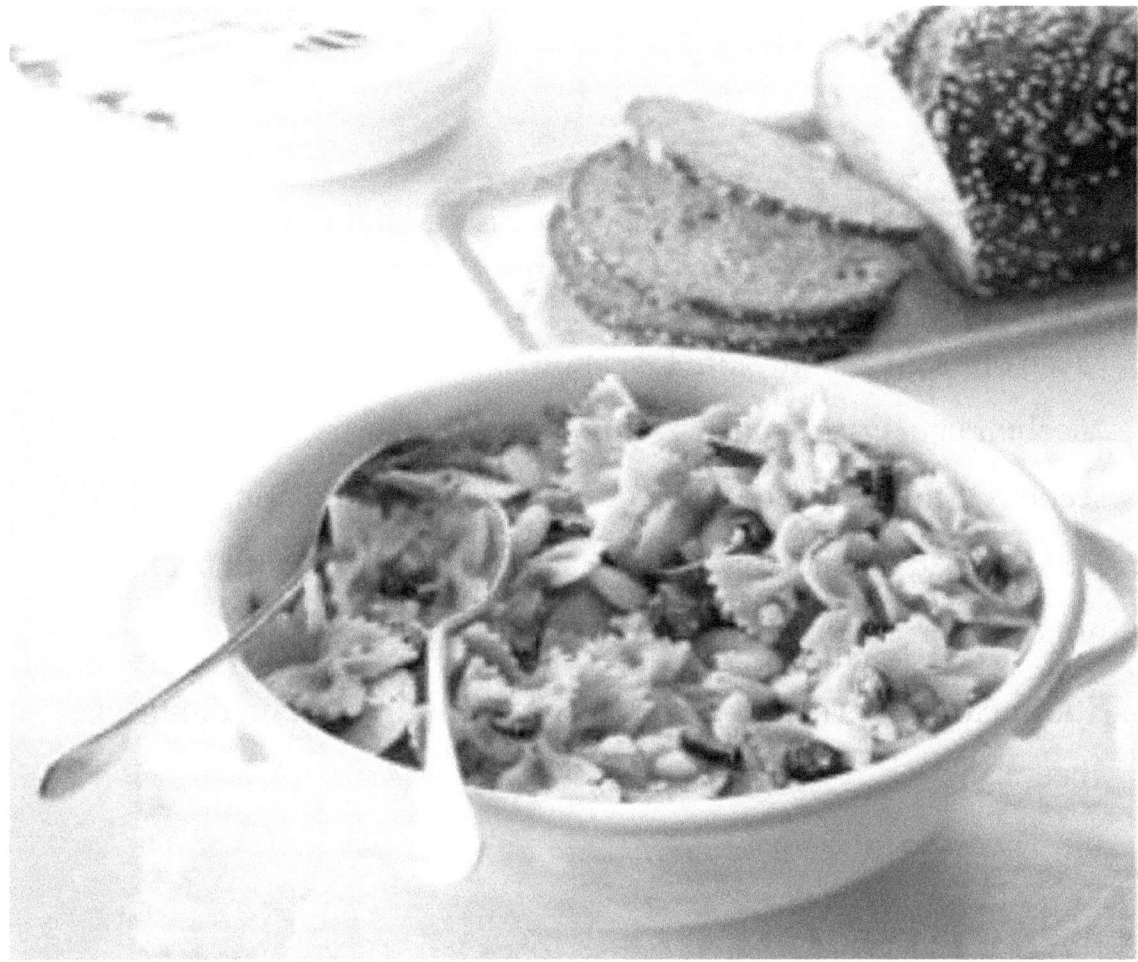

Prep Time: 5 mins
Cook Time: 20 mins
Total Time: 25 min.
Servings: 4

Ingredients

- ☐ 2-1/2 cups uncooked whole wheat bow tie pasta (about 6 ounces)
- ☐ 1 tablespoon olive oil
- ☐ 1 medium zucchini, sliced
- ☐ 2 garlic cloves, minced
- ☐ 2 large tomatoes, chopped (about 2-1/2 cups)
- ☐ 1 can (15 ounces) cannellini beans, rinsed and drained
- ☐ 1 can (2-1/4 ounces) sliced ripe olives, drained

☐ 3/4 teaspoon freshly ground pepper

☐ 1/2 cup crumbled feta cheese

Directions

1. Cook pasta according to package directions. Drain, reserving 1/2 cup pasta water.

2. Meanwhile, in a large skillet, heat oil over medium-high heat; saute zucchini until crisp-tender, 2-4 minutes. Add garlic; cook and stir 30 seconds. Stir in tomatoes, beans, olives and pepper; bring to a boil. Reduce heat; simmer, uncovered, until tomatoes are softened, 3-5 minutes, stirring occasionally.

3. Stir in pasta and enough pasta water to moisten as desired. Stir in cheese.

29. Garden Vegetable Beef Soup

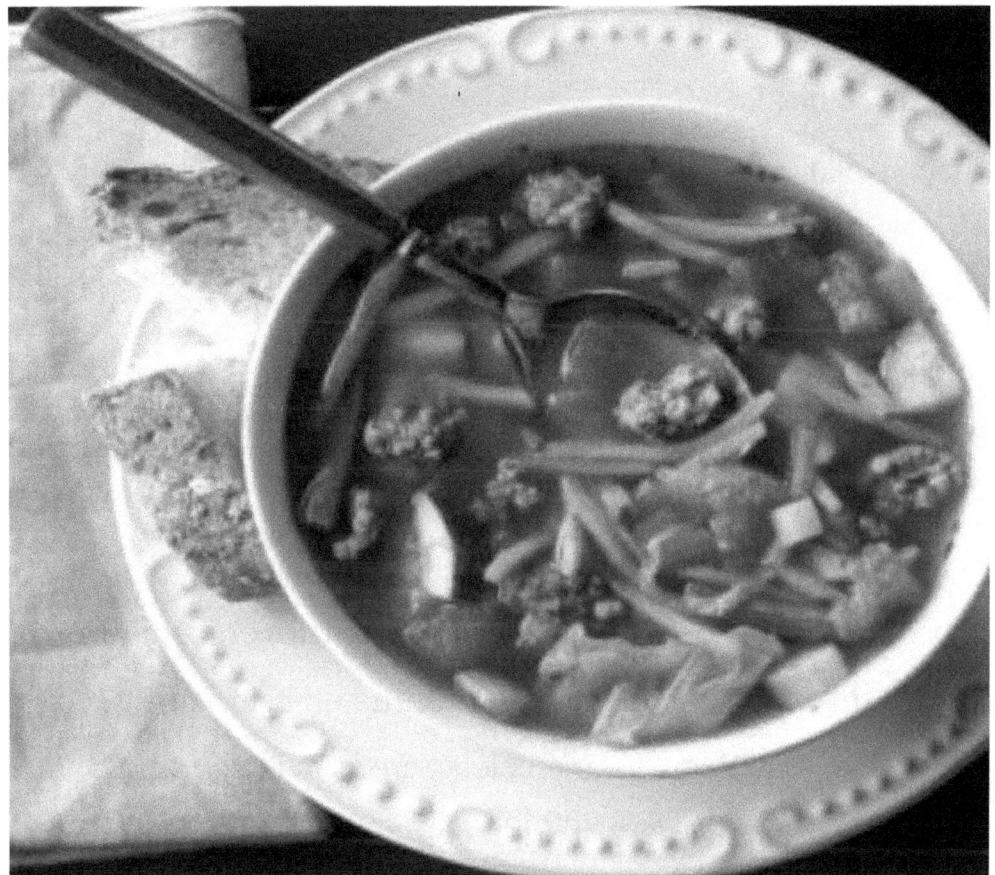

Prep Time: 20 mins
Cook Time: 55 mins
Total Time: 1 hr 15 mins
Servings: 8

Ingredients

- ☐ 1-1/2 pounds lean ground beef (90% lean)
- ☐ 1 medium onion, chopped
- ☐ 2 garlic cloves, minced
- ☐ 1 package (10 ounces) julienned carrots
- ☐ 2 celery ribs, chopped
- ☐ 1/4 cup tomato paste
- ☐ 1 can (14-1/2 ounces) diced tomatoes, undrained
- ☐ 1-1/2 cups shredded cabbage
- ☐ 1 medium zucchini, coarsely chopped

- [ ] 1 medium red potato (about 5 ounces), finely chopped
- [ ] 1/2 cup fresh or frozen cut green beans
- [ ] 1 teaspoon dried basil
- [ ] 1/2 teaspoon dried oregano
- [ ] 1/4 teaspoon salt
- [ ] 1/4 teaspoon pepper
- [ ] 4 cans (14-1/2 ounces each) reduced-sodium beef broth
- [ ] Grated Parmesan cheese, optional

Directions

1. In a large bowl, cook the beef with onion and garlic over medium heat 6-8 minutes or till beef is no longer pink, cutting up beef into smaller parts; drain. Put together carrots and celery; cook and keep stirring it up to 6-8 minutes or until tender. Turn together the tomato paste; cook 1 minute again.

2. Put tomatoes, cabbage, zucchini, potato, green beans, seasonings and broth; bring to a boil. Minimize the heat; simmer, covered, 35-45 minutes or till the vegetables are soften. If like, top each serving with cheese.

30. Raspberry Peach Puff Pancake

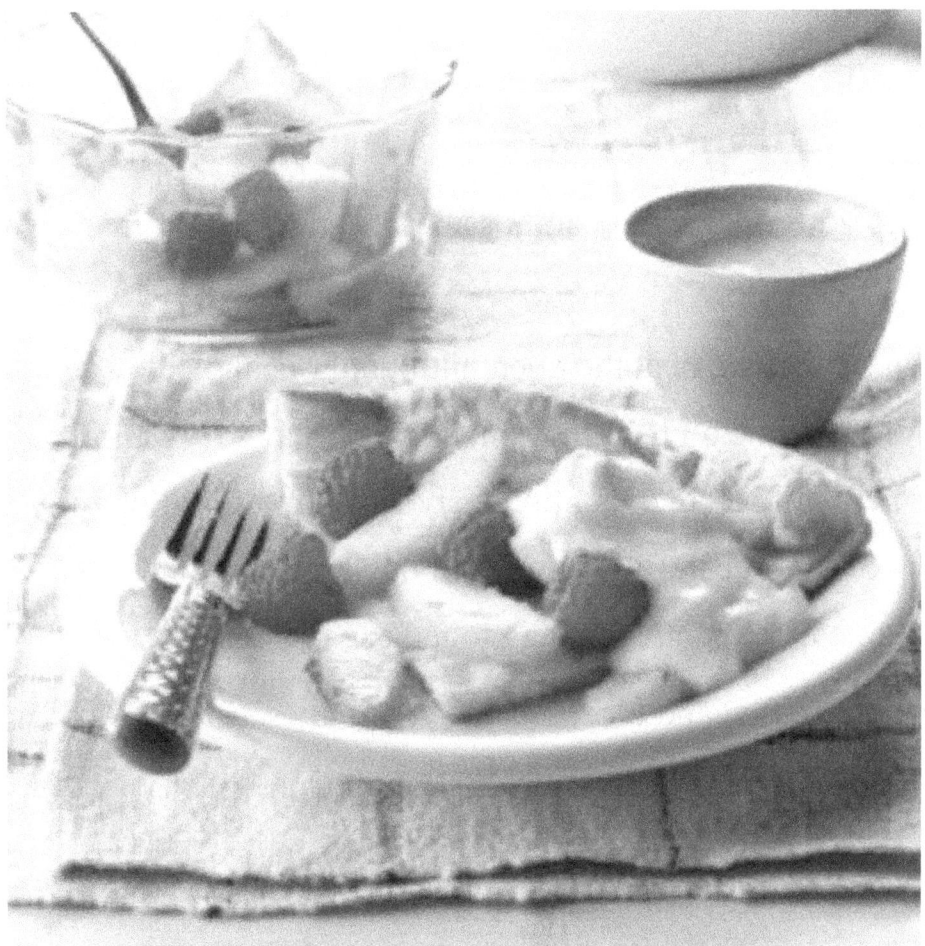

Prep Time: 15 mins
Cook Time: 20 mins
Total Time: 35 mins
Servings: 4

Ingredients

- ☐ 2 medium peaches, peeled and sliced
- ☐ 1/2 teaspoon sugar
- ☐ 1/2 cup fresh raspberries
- ☐ 1 tablespoon butter
- ☐ 3 large eggs, lightly beaten
- ☐ 1/2 cup fat-free milk
- ☐ 1/8 teaspoon salt

- ☐ 1/2 cup all-purpose flour
- ☐ 1/4 cup vanilla yoghurt

Directions

1. Preheat oven to 400°. In a small pan, toss peaches; gently stir in raspberries.

2. Place butter in a 9-in pan; heat the oven until butter is melted on at least 2-3 minutes. While on that, in a small skillet, whisk eggs, milk and salt together until blended; continuously whisk in flour. Put away pie plate from oven; tilt carefully to coat on the down part and sides with butter. Immediately put in the egg together.

3. Bake until cake is puffed and browned, 18-22 minutes. Put away from oven; serve immediately with fruit and yoghurt.

31. Breakfast Fruit Pizzas

Prep Time: 10mins
Cook Time: 2mins
Total Time: 12mins
Servings: 4

Ingredients

- ☐ 2whole-wheat pita flatbreads
- ☐ 7ouncesArla Original Cream Cheese
- ☐ 1-2teaspoonshoney
- ☐ 1/2teaspoonpure vanilla extract
- ☐ 3kiwiskin removed and sliced
- ☐ 1/2cupsliced strawberries
- ☐ 1/2cupblackberries
- ☐ 1/4cupblueberries
- ☐ 2raspberriesfor the centre

Directions

1. Preheat oven to broil. Place the whole wheat pita flatbreads in the oven, directly on the rack. Broil for 1 minute and flip. Broil for another minute. You can also toast the bread in a toaster oven or toaster if your toaster is large enough. Set the bread aside to cool.

2. In a small bowl, stir together the cream cheese, honey, and vanilla. Spread the cream cheese on the pita bread.

3. Arrange the fruit on top of the cream cheese. Get creative and decorate the pizzas however you like! Cut into slices and serve immediately.

4. Note-you can use your favourite fruit. Bananas, peaches, pineapple, oranges, nectarines would also be good!

32. Wedge Salad Skewers

Prep Time:10mins
Total Time:10mins
Servings:8

Ingredients

- ☐ 1head of iceberg lettuce(cut into wedge pieces)
- ☐ 4Roma tomatoes cut in half
- ☐ 1red onion(cut into 1-inch pieces)
- ☐ 2avocados cut into 1-inch pieces
- ☐ 5piecesof bacon cooked and cut into thirds
- ☐ 1cucumber(sliced (peeled or unpeeled))
- ☐ 8wooden skewers
- ☐ 2green onions(diced)
- ☐ 1 5ozcontainer blue cheese crumbles
- ☐ 1bottle blue cheese dressing

Directions

1. One skewer at a time adds an iceberg wedge, tomato, onion, avocado, two pieces of bacon, another iceberg wedge and then cucumber.

2. Continue until all skewers have been made then garnish with crumbled blue cheese, blue cheese dressing, and diced green onions.

33. Southwestern Brown Rice Bowl

Prep Time: 10 mins
Cook Time: 20 mins
Total Time: 30 mins
Servings: 4

Ingredients

For the Rice:

- ☐ 2cupsbrown rice
- ☐ 1shallotroughly chopped
- ☐ 2cupstightly packed fresh cilantro leavestough stems removed
- ☐ 1clovegarlic
- ☐ 1/2teaspoonsred pepper flakes
- ☐ 1/2cupolive oil
- ☐ 2tablespoonsred wine vinegar
- ☐ 1teaspoonsalt

For the Toppings:

- ☐ Black Beans
- ☐ 1recipe Guacamole
- ☐ Pico dc Gallorecipe below
- ☐ Shredded Romaine Lettuce
- ☐ Chopped yellow or orange bell peppers
- ☐ Freshly Shredded Colby Jack Cheese
- ☐ Additional cilantro for garnish

For the Pico de Gallo

- ☐ 1 1/2poundsripe tomatoescut into 1/4- to 1/2-inch dice
- ☐ Kosher salt
- ☐ 1/2large white onionfinely diced (about 3/4 cup)
- ☐ 1 to 2jalapeño chillies finely diced (seeds and membranes removed for a milder salsa)

- ☐ 1/2cupfinely chopped fresh cilantro leaves
- ☐ 1tablespoonlime juice from 1 lime

Directions

1. Cook the brown rice in a rice cooker according to the package directions

2. Bring together all the ingredients for the cilantro vinaigrette in a high quality blender and blend for 60 seconds until very soft. Taste it and add little salt if possible and pepper as needed. Fold the vinaigrette into the cooked brown rice.

3. Divide the rice amongst 4 bowls and top with black beans, guacamole, pico de gallo, shredded lettuce, bell peppers and cheese. Add extra cilantro to garnish if desired

34. Low Sodium Sheet Pan Chicken Fajitas

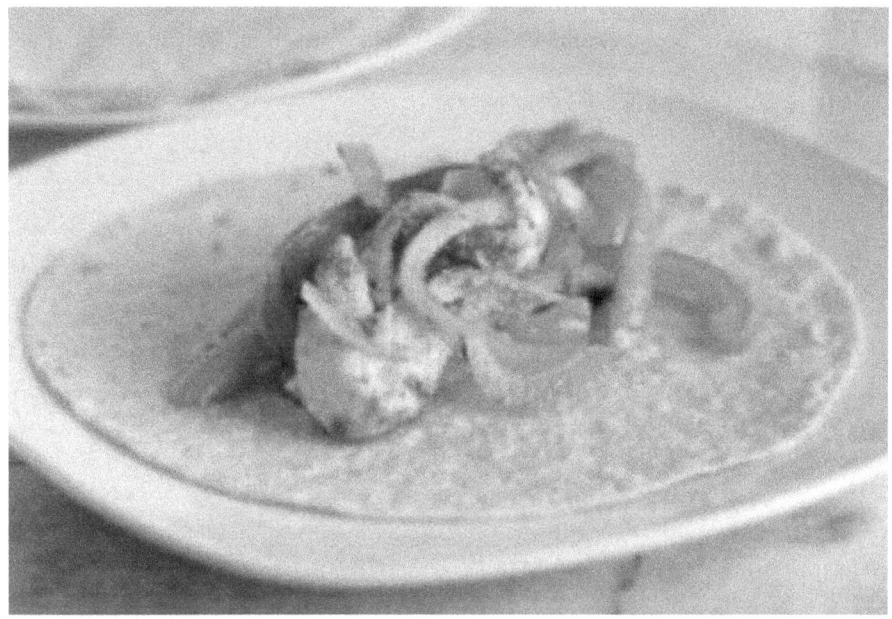

Prep Time:5mins
Cook Time: 20mins
Total Time: 25mins
Servings: 8

Ingredients

- [ ] 2lbschicken breast tenderloineach sliced in half lengthwise
- [ ] 1green peppersliced
- [ ] 1red bell peppersliced
- [ ] 1Vidalia onionsliced

Olive oil spray

- [ ] 1tablespoonolive oil

Seasoning:

- [ ] 1teaspoonchilli powder
- [ ] 1/2teaspoonsmoked paprika
- [ ] 1/2teaspoongarlic powder
- [ ] 1/2teaspoononion powder
- [ ] 1/2teaspoondried oregano

☐ 1/2teaspoondried cilantro

☐ 1/2teaspooncumin

☐ 1/4teaspooncayenne pepper

Directions

1. Preheat oven to 350 degrees F.
2. Coat a sheet pan with olive oil spray.
3. Spread pepper and onion slices onto a prepared sheet pan.
4. Place chicken slices on top of vegetables.
5. Combine seasoning ingredients and stir to combine.
6. Sprinkle seasoning mixture over chicken, peppers, and onion.
7. Drizzle 1 tablespoon of olive oil over chicken, peppers, and onion.
8. Gently toss ingredients to evenly distribute seasoning and oil. (make sure chicken strips are not overlapping)
9. Bake for 20 minutes or until chicken reaches 165 degrees F.
10. Serve in warm low sodium tortillas.
11. Top with your favourite toppings! I love cheddar cheese and sour cream.

35. Turkish Red Lentil Soup

Prep Time: 15mins
Cook Time:45mins
Total Time: 1 hr
Servings: 4

Ingredients

For a large pan of Red Lentil Soup

- ☐ 1 large onion (or 2 medium) — White or Red
- ☐ 3 large cloves of Garlic
- ☐ 5 medium-large Carrots
- ☐ 2 sticks of Celery
- ☐ 5 large teaspoons of Tomato concentrate/ paste
- ☐ 500g of Red Lentils
- ☐ Chicken stock to fill your pan
- ☐ 1 heaped tablespoon of dried mint
- ☐ 1 heaped tablespoon of dried Oregano
- ☐ Olive Oil, Salt and Black Pepper

Directions

1. You can, of course, use ready Chicken Stock but we like to make our own as a good stock will enhance your soup. If there is any leftover carcass from the roast chicken, then this is an excellent thrifty alternative. We make use of some fresh chicken pieces like 3 thighs. Put it in your pan, fill 2/3 with chilled water and put on the heat. If there are any vegetable off cuts from Onions, Carrots, Celery, Leeks or a couple of Bay leaves etc. Add these in to the flavor. When the stock is beginning to simmer, reduce the heat, so it simmers softly for at least an hour. For a Vegetarian/ Vegan they can use any alternative.

2. Meanwhile easily chop your vegetables. A food processor is needed. Soften these in a medium pan with a good quality Olive Oil. Cook gently until the vegetable is soft and the natural good and enhanced. Put together your Tomato, season with little Salt and Pepper and cook for another 5 minutes.

3. When your stock is ready for use, set aside the chicken pieces and leave to cool down. If the chicken has calm, it's safest to strain the stock for any small piece you want.

4. Clean your Lentils and put together with the stock and softened vegetables in a large pan. Add all your herbs. Well prepared to taste but do not over-Salt as the flavors will be on the cooking. Cook together on a easy simmer for 2 hours until the Lentils are just begin to break down.

36. Chickpea Brownies

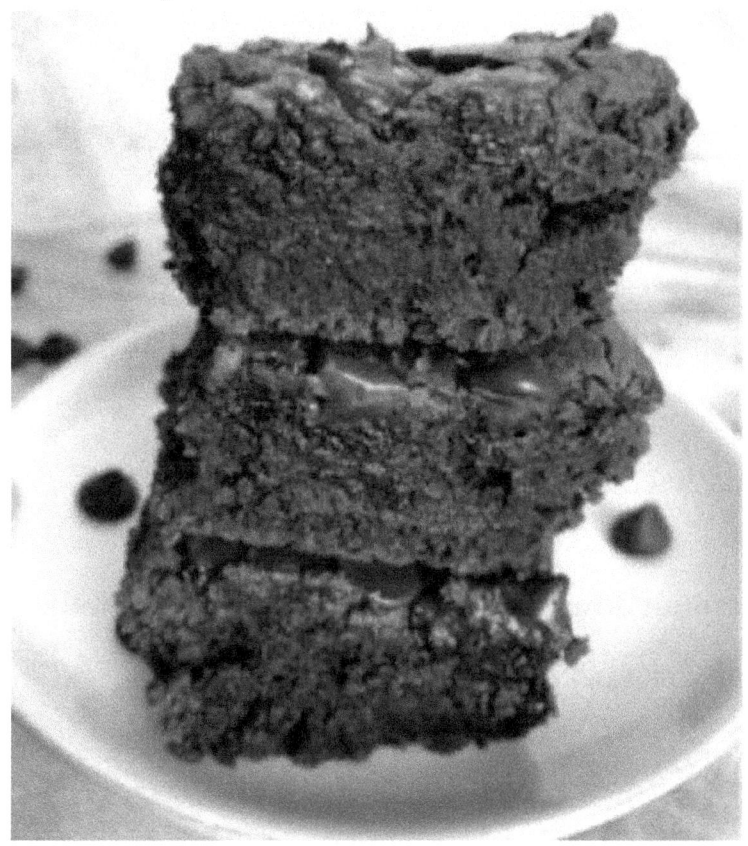

Prep Time:5mins
Cook Time:20mins
Total Time:25 mins
Servings: 4

Ingredients

- ☐ 1 – 15oz can chickpeas, drained and rinsed.

- ☐ 1/2 cup nut butter (I like almond or peanut)

- ☐ 1/2 cup maple syrup

- ☐ 1 Tbsp melted coconut oil

- ☐ 1 tsp. vanilla

- ☐ 1/4 cup almond flour

- ☐ 1/4 cup cocoa powder

- ☐ 1/4 tsp baking soda

- ☐ 1/4 tsp baking powder
- ☐ 1/4 tsp salt
- ☐ 1/2 cup chocolate chips and more for sprinkling on top!

Directions

1. Preheat oven to 350F.
2. In a large pan blend the chickpeas, butter nut; this will bring about the well needed taste.
3. Once blended, add in almond flour, cocoa powder, baking soda, baking powder, and salt.
4. Continue to process, scraping down sides as necessary until smooth.
5. Once creamy and smooth, take off the lid (I also remove blade) and stir in chocolate chips.
6. Do not process the chips.
7. Pour into greased 8×8 pan and sprinkle with extra chocolate chips if desired. see note for extra thickness
8. Bake for 21-23 minutes.

37. Blackened Chicken with Berry Salad

Prep Time:15 mins
Cook Time:15 mins
Total Time:30 mins
Servings:2

Ingredients

- ☐ 2 4 oz chicken breast
- ☐ Cherry tomatoes
- ☐ 1 tbsp Cajun spice
- ☐ 4 ounces crumbled blue cheese
- ☐ 6 ounces of your favourite salad greens
- ☐ 1 peach (fresh)
- ☐ Cooking spray
- ☐ For the dressing:
- ☐ 1 lemon
- ☐ 1 lime
- ☐ 1/4 C brown sugar
- ☐ 2 tbsp mustard (Dijon or whole grain)
- ☐ 1 tsp chopped garlic
- ☐ 1/2 C olive oil
- ☐ 1/4 C white balsamic vinegar

Directions

1. Heat a cast-iron skillet until super hot.

2. Sprinkle Cajun spice over chicken breast until thoroughly coated.

3. Place chicken in skillet and cook for 4-5 minutes (do not use any oil in the pan).

4. Turn chicken over and cook additional 4-5 minutes.

5. This may smoke a lot, so do this in the kitchen that is well-ventilated.

6. Remove chicken from pan and let rest while preparing the dressing.

7. To grill peaches:

8. Slice into wedges and spray with cooking spray and place on a medium-high grill for 1 to 2 minutes per side. Remove and allow to cool at room temperature for 3-4 minutes.

9. In a mixing bowl juice the lemon and lime, add the, garlic, and mustard and mix together.

10.   Add vinegar and while whisking slowly drizzle the olive oil in the mixture until well combined.

11.   To assemble salad:

12.   Place greens on a plate, top with crumbled blue cheese, cherry tomatoes, grilled peaches and sliced carrots.

13.   Slice chicken breast and top salad.

14.   Drizzle dressing over the top and enjoy.

38. Tuna Salad Plate

Prep Time: 10mins
Total Time: 10mins
Servings: 4

Ingredients

- ☐ 25 ounce canstuna in waterdrained
- ☐ 1/4cupplain Greek yoghurtor mayonnaise, plus more as desired
- ☐ 2tablespoonsrelish
- ☐ 2tablespoonsfinely chopped red onionor to taste
- ☐ 2tablespoonschopped celery
- ☐ salt and pepperto taste

Directions

1. Put in the drained tuna in a medium pan.

2. Add the plain Greek yoghurt (or mayonnaise), relish, red onion, celery, and a little salt and pepper.

3. Stir with a fork until everything is well combined. Taste it and add salt if needed and pepper as needed too.

4. Serve tuna salad on bread, rolls, croissants or crackers. If you needed a low carb, serving a good tuna salad on a bed of lettuce, in hollowed out tomatoes, or in avocado halves are always the best.

39. Frittatas

Prep Time:20 minutes
Cook Time:25 minutes
Total Time:45 minutes
Servings : 8

Ingredients

- ☐ 12 eggs
- ☐ 3 tablespoons full-fat dairy (heavy cream, half-and-half, whole milk, sour cream, crème fraîche or yoghurt)
- ☐ ½ teaspoon salt
- ☐ 1 cup (4 ounces) grated or crumbled cheese
- ☐ 3 to 5 cups vegetables or greens of choice (or 3 cups leftover cooked vegetables or greens)
- ☐ 1 tablespoon olive oil
- ☐ Garnish: Chopped or torn fresh, leafy herbs (basil, parsley, cilantro, or dill)

Directions

1. Preheat the oven to 425 degrees Fahrenheit for the traditional stovetop method, or 350 degrees for the baked methods (casserole or mini/muffins).

2. Break the eggs into a medium mixing pan. Add your dairy of your choice and the salt. Whisk just until the egg yolks and whites are blended. Whisk all the cheese (you can reserve the other half for topping the frittata before baking if you prefer). Set the mixture aside.

3. Warm the olive oil in a 12″ cast iron skillet or oven-safe non-stick skillet until shimmering. Add the vegetables, starting with chopped onions or other dense vegetables. Cook for a few minutes, stirring occasionally, and then add any softer vegetables such as zucchini.

Keep cooking until those vegetables are soft and tender, then add any garlic or greens, and cook until the aroma or wilted. Season with salt, to taste.

4. Traditional stovetop option: Whisk the eggs once more and pour the mixture over the vegetables. Stir with a spatula briefly to combine and distribute the mixture evenly across the pan. If there is any left over any cheese, spray it on top of the frittata now.

5. Once the outside edge of the frittata turns lighter in colour (about 30 seconds to 1 minute), carefully transfer the frittata to the oven. Bake for 7 to 14 minutes (keep an eye on it), until the eggs are puffed and appear cooked, and the centre of the frittata jiggles just a bit when you give it a gentle shimmy. Remove the frittata from the oven and place it on a cooling rack to cool. Garnish with vegetable, slice with a sharp knife, it's ready to serve.

6. Baked casserole option: Let the cooked vegetables cool for a few minutes, and then stir them into the egg mixture. On a large skillet, and then pour the mixed items together into the skillet. If there is any leftover cheese, sprinkle it on top of the frittata now.

7. Bake for 20 to 25 minutes (keep an eye on it), until the eggs are puffed and appear cooked, and the centre of the frittata jiggles just a bit when you give it a gentle shimmy. Remove the frittata from the oven and place it on a cooling rack to cool. Garnish with vegetables, slice with a sharp knife, and serve.

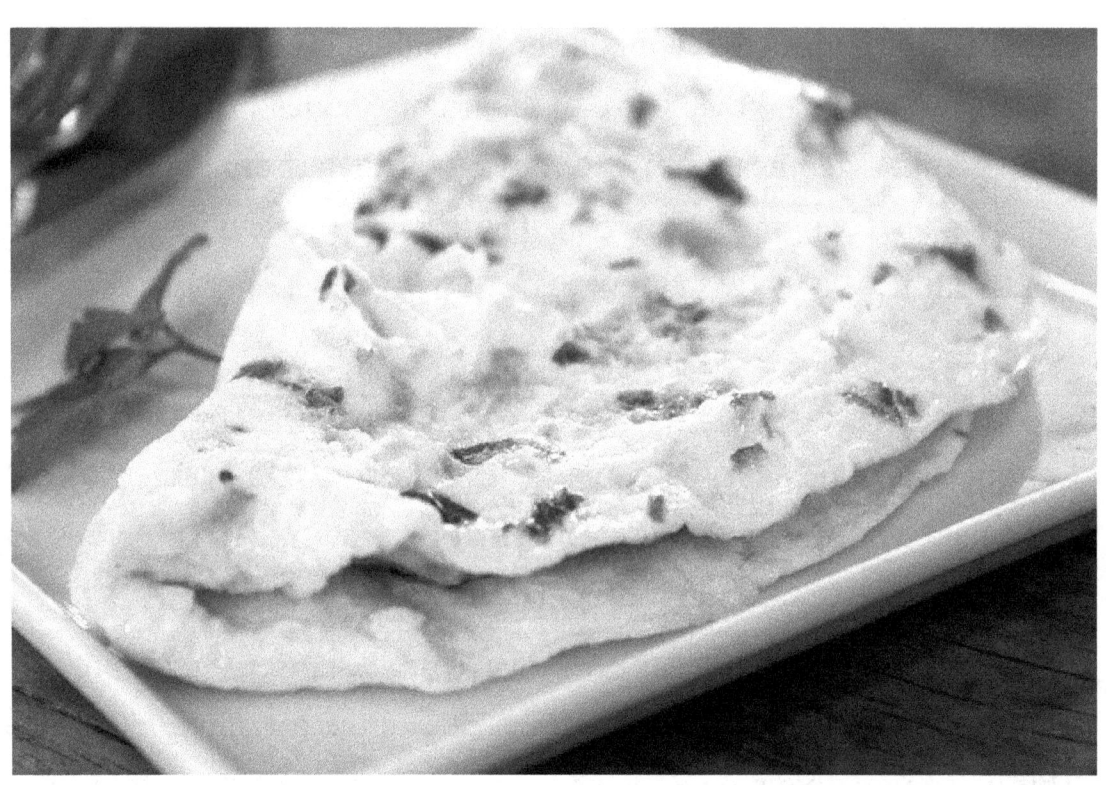

40.Spaghetti Squash with Meaty Sauce

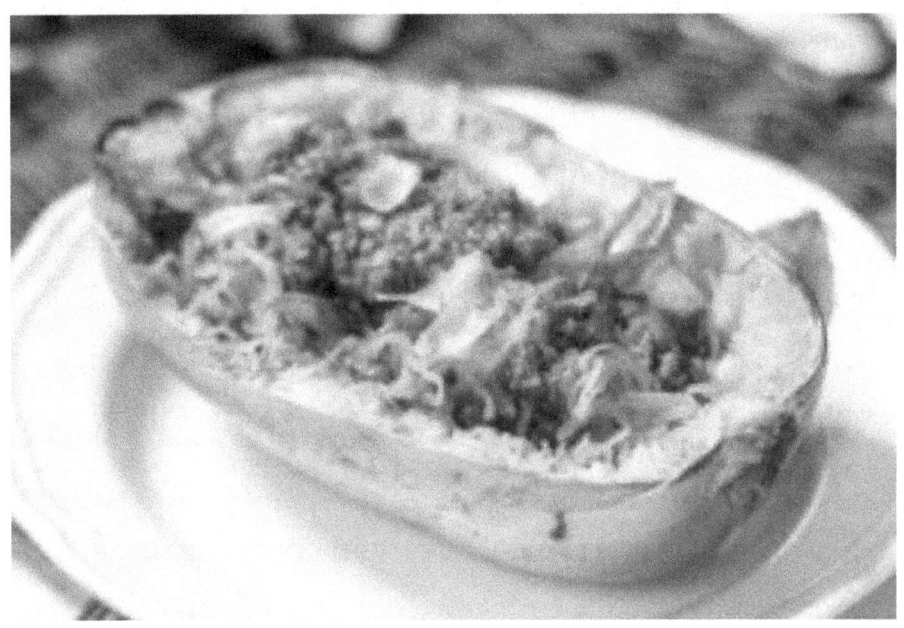

Prep time: 15 mins
Cook time: 55 mins
Total time: 1 hour 10 mins
Servings: 4

Ingredients

- ☐ 3 tablespoons olive oil, divided
- ☐ 2 (3 lb) spaghetti squash, sliced in half lengthwise, seeds removed
- ☐ 1.5 pounds ground beef
- ☐ 1 medium yellow onion, finely diced
- ☐ 2 medium carrots, peeled, and grated
- ☐ 2 cloves garlic, minced
- ☐ 1 can (28 ounces) crushed tomatoes + a little water
- ☐ ½ teaspoon crushed red pepper flakes
- ☐ ½ cup grated Parmesan Cheese, divided, plus more for topping
- ☐ Fresh basil leaves, cut into thin ribbons or left whole
- ☐ Salt and pepper to taste

Directions

1. Preheat oven to 400F.

2. Place the spaghetti squash halves cut side up onto a baking sheet. Drizzle with only 1 tsp of olive oil divide together with salt, and pepper. Put on the squash over so they're cut side down, and roast properly for 50-60 minutes, or until a knife can pierces into the thickest part of the squash ea freely. Strands should be tender, but shouldn't be mushy. Allow it to cool for 10 minutes. Once cooled enough to handle, use a fork to remove the squash strands, right in their shells. Drizzle the strands carefully with 1 tsp of olive oil, salt, pepper, and the Parmesan Cheese well mixed.

3. While the squash is cooking, in a large pan or wide pot, heat the remaining tablespoon of olive oil over high. Include beef and cook by breaking it up, until it begins to color, about 5 minutes. Add onion, carrots, and garlic and season with salt and pepper. Keep cooking until the vegetables are tender, about 5 minutes. Add the crushed tomatoes and red pepper flakes. Add a little water to the can and swish out all the goodies too. Bring to a rapid simmer.

4. Cover and let it continue to cook for 15 minutes, stirring occasionally, until the liquid is slightly reduced and the flavors are melded. Taste and season with salt and pepper. Serve the sauce together with spaghetti squash, right in their shells, and one-half shell per person.

41. Shrimp & Nectarine Salad

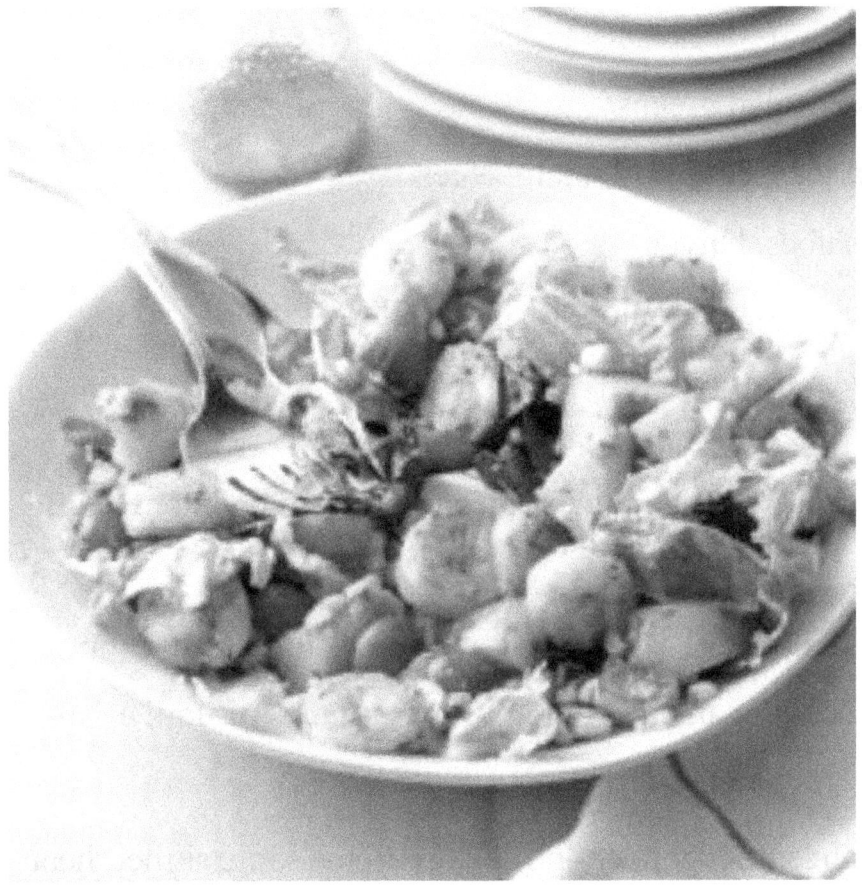

Prep Time: 10 mins
Cook Time: 20 mins
Total Time: 30 min
Servings : 4

Ingredients

- ☐ 1/3 cup orange juice
- ☐ 3 tablespoons cider vinegar
- ☐ 1-1/2 teaspoons Dijon mustard
- ☐ 1-1/2 teaspoons honey
- ☐ 1 tablespoon minced fresh tarragon

SALAD:

- ☐ 4 teaspoons canola oil, divided
- ☐ 1 cup fresh or frozen corn
- ☐ 1 pound uncooked shrimp (26-30 per pound), peeled and deveined

- ☐ 1/2 teaspoon lemon-pepper seasoning
- ☐ 1/4 teaspoon salt
- ☐ 8 cups torn mixed salad greens
- ☐ 2 medium nectarines, cut into 1-inch pieces
- ☐ 1 cup grape tomatoes, halved
- ☐ 1/2 cup finely chopped red onion

Directions

1. In a small bowl, whisk orange juice, vinegar, mustard and honey until blended. Stir in tarragon.

2. With a medium skillet, heat 1 tsp oil over medium-high heat. Input your corn; keep cooking and stirring until 1-2 minutes or until crisp-soft. Keep away from pan.

3. Spray shrimp with lemon, pepper and salt. With the same skillet, heat left over oil over medium-high heat. Put together shrimp; cook and stir 3-4 minutes or till you see shrimp turn pink. Stir in corn.

4. With a large pan, combine left over ingredients. Drizzle with 1/3 cup dressing and toss to coat it. Separate the mixture among four plates. Add with shrimp mixture; drizzle with left over dressing. Serve warm.

42. Pork Chops with Tomato Curry

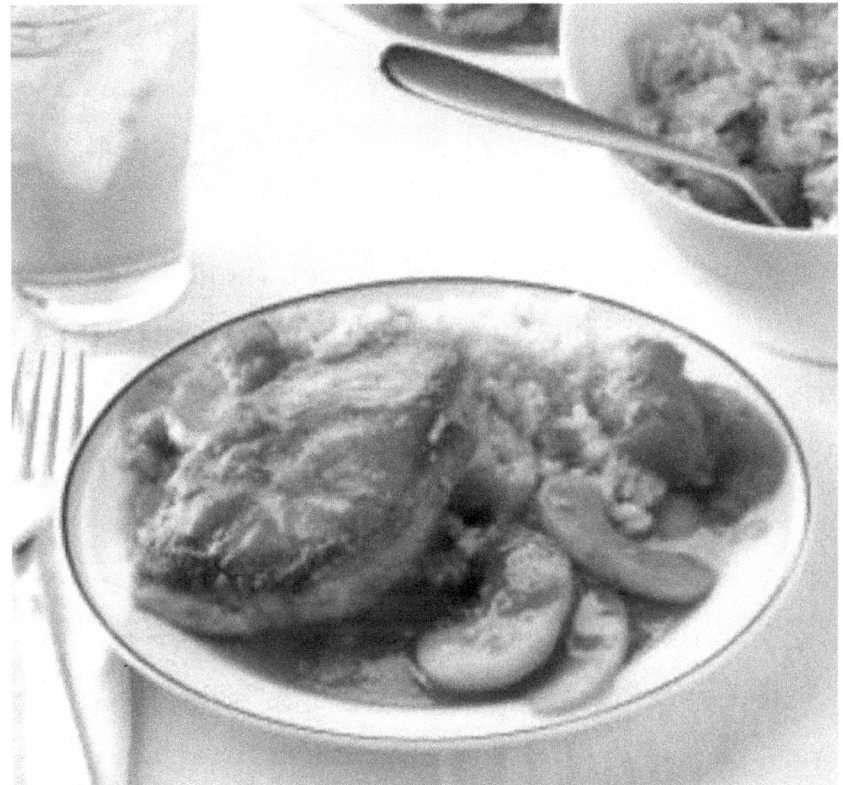

Prep Time: 15 mins
Cook Time: 25 mins
Total Time: 40 mins
Servings : 6

Ingredients

- ☐ 4 teaspoons butter, divided
- ☐ 6 boneless pork loin chops (6 ounces each)
- ☐ 1 small onion, finely chopped
- ☐ 3 medium apples, thinly sliced (about 5 cups)
- ☐ 1 can (28 ounces) whole tomatoes, undrained
- ☐ 4 teaspoons sugar
- ☐ 2 teaspoons curry powder
- ☐ 1/2 teaspoon salt
- ☐ 1/2 teaspoon chili powder
- ☐ 4 cups hot cooked brown rice

☐   2 tablespoons toasted slivered almonds, optional

Directions

1. In a 6-qt. stockpot, heat 2 teaspoons butter over medium-high heat. Brown pork chops in batches. Remove from pan.

2. In same pan, heat remaining butter over medium heat. Include onions; keep cooking and stirring 2-3 minutes or until softened. Keep turning the apples, tomatoes, sugar, curry powder, salt and chili powder. Gather to a boil, stirring consciously to break up tomatoes.

3. Return chops to pan. Reduce heat; simmer, uncovered, 5 minutes. Keep turning chops; cook it up to 3-5 minutes longer or until a thermometer inserted in pork are reads 145°. Allow it cool for 5 minutes minimum before serving. Serve with rice and, if desired, sprinkle with almonds.

43. Overnight Oatmeal

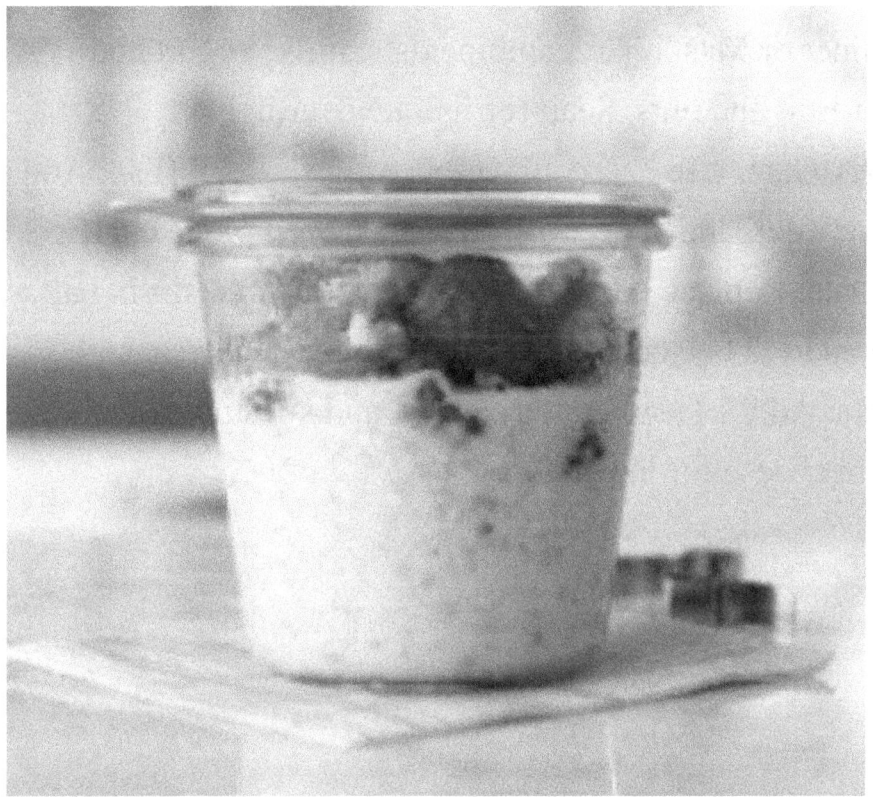

Prep Time: 10 min. + chilling

Total Time: 10

Servings: 6

Ingredients

- ☐ 1/3 cup old-fashioned oats
- ☐ 3 tablespoons fat-free milk
- ☐ 3 tablespoons reduced-fat plain yogurt
- ☐ 1 tablespoon honey
- ☐ 1/2 cup assorted fresh fruit
- ☐ 2 tablespoons chopped walnuts, toasted

Directions

1. In a small container or Mason jar, combine oats, milk, yogurt and honey. Top with fruit and nuts. Seal; refrigerate overnight.
2. Chocolate-Cherry Oats: Use cherry-flavored yogurt; add 1 Tbsp. Add together cocoa powder, and spray with fresh or frozen pitted cherries.
3. Banana Bread Oats: Replace honey with maple syrup and stir in half a mashed banana and 1/2 tsp. cinnamon. Top with toasted pecans.
4. Carrot Cake Oats: Add 2 Tbsp. grated carrots, and substitute spreadable cream cheese for the yogurt.

44. Thai Chicken Pasta Skillet

Total Time: 10 mins

Cook Time: 20 mins

Total Time: 30 mins.

Servings: 6

Ingredients

- ☐ 6 ounces uncooked whole wheat spaghetti
- ☐ 2 teaspoons canola oil
- ☐ 1 package (10 ounces) fresh sugar snap peas, trimmed and cut diagonally into thin strips
- ☐ 2 cups julienned carrots (about 8 ounces)
- ☐ 2 cups shredded cooked chicken
- ☐ 1 cup Thai peanut sauce
- ☐ 1 medium cucumber, halved lengthwise, seeded and sliced diagonally
- ☐ Chopped fresh cilantro, optional

Directions

1. Cook pasta consistent with package directions; drain.
2. Meanwhile, in a very giant frying pan, heat oil over medium-high heat. Add snap peas and carrots; stir-fry 6-8 minutes or till crisp-tender. Add chicken, peanut sauce and spaghetti; heat through, moving to mix.
3. Transfer to a serving plate. high with cucumber and, if desired, cilantro.

45. Chili-Lime Grilled Pineapple

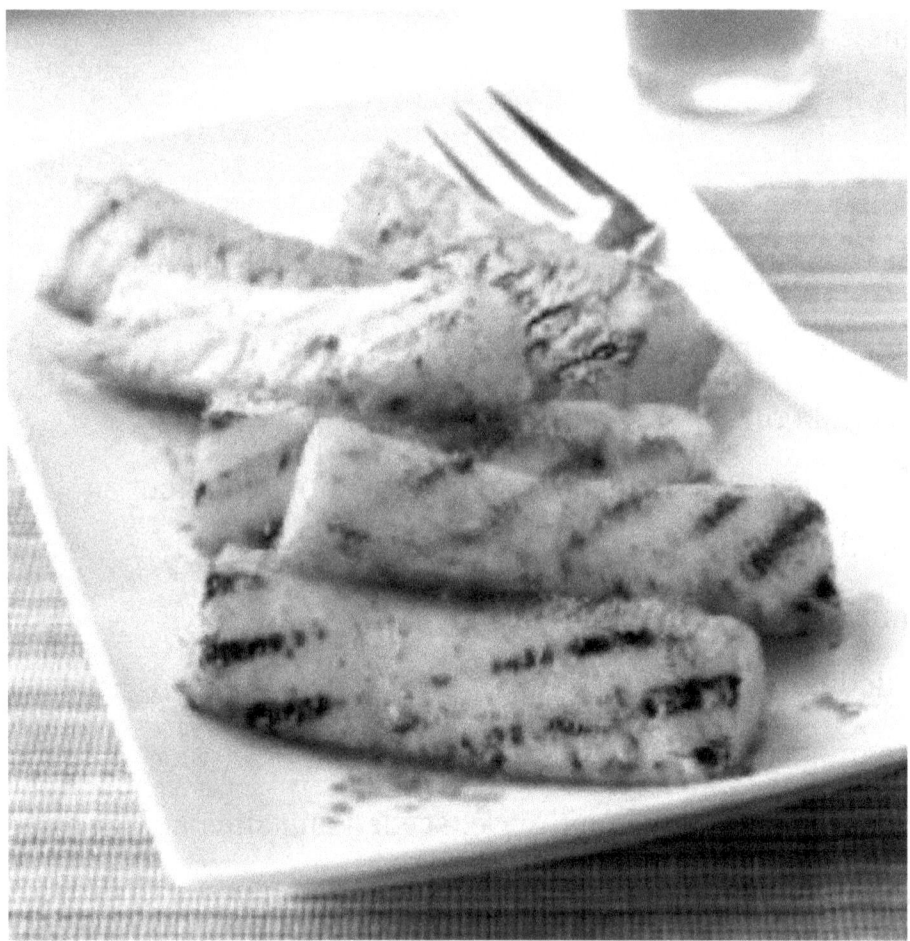

Prep Time: 5 mins

Cook Time: 10 mins

Total Time: 15 mins.

Servings: 6

Ingredients

- [ ] 1 fresh pineapple
- [ ] 3 tablespoons brown sugar
- [ ] 1 tablespoon lime juice
- [ ] 1 tablespoon olive oil
- [ ] 1 tablespoon honey or agave nectar
- [ ] 1-1/2 teaspoons chili powder
- [ ] Dash salt

Directions

1. Peel pineapple, removing any eyes from fruit. Cut lengthwise into vi wedges; take away core. in a very little bowl, combine remaining ingredients till blended . Brush pineapple with half the glaze; reserve remaining mixture for basting.

2. Grill pineapple, covered, over medium heat or broil 4 in. from heat 2-4 minutes on each side or until lightly browned, basting occasionally with reserved glaze.

46. Italian Sausage-Stuffed Zucchini

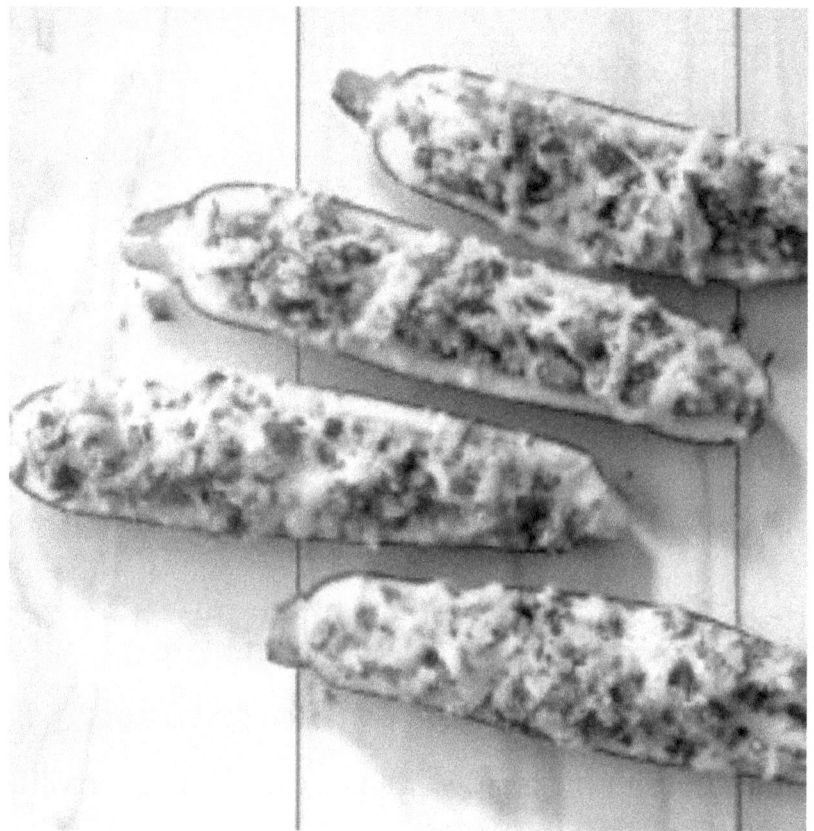

Prep Time: 35 mins.
Cook Time: 20 mins.
Total Time: 55 mins
Servings : 6

Ingredients

- ☐ 6 medium zucchini (about 8 ounces each)
- ☐ 1 pound Italian turkey sausage links, casings removed
- ☐ 2 medium tomatoes, seeded and chopped
- ☐ 1 cup panko (Japanese) bread crumbs
- ☐ 1/3 cup grated Parmesan cheese
- ☐ 1/3 cup minced fresh parsley
- ☐ 2 tablespoons minced fresh oregano or 2 teaspoons dried oregano
- ☐ 2 tablespoons minced fresh basil or 2 teaspoons dried basil
- ☐ 1/4 teaspoon pepper

- ☐ 3/4 cup shredded part-skim mozzarella cheese
- ☐ Additional minced fresh parsley, optional

Directions

1. Heat oven to 350°. Put in the zucchini in half. Remove out pulp, leaving a 1/4-in. shell; chop pulp. Add on the zucchini shells in a larger microwave-safe box. In batches, microwave, covered, on high 2-3 minutes or till crisp-tender.

2. Put in a large skillet, continue cooking sausage and zucchini pulp over medium heat 6-8 minutes or till the sausage is no longer pink, before breaking sausage into crumbles; keep stirring in tomatoes, bread crumbs, Parmesan cheese, vegetables and pepper. Spoon into zucchini shells.

3. Place in 2 ungreased 13x9-in. baking dishes. Cover and bake up to 15-20 minutes or until zucchini is tender. Top up with mozzarella cheese. Bake, cover it very well up to 5-8 minutes longer or until cheese is melted. If desired, sprinkle with additional minced parsley.

47. Spicy Almonds

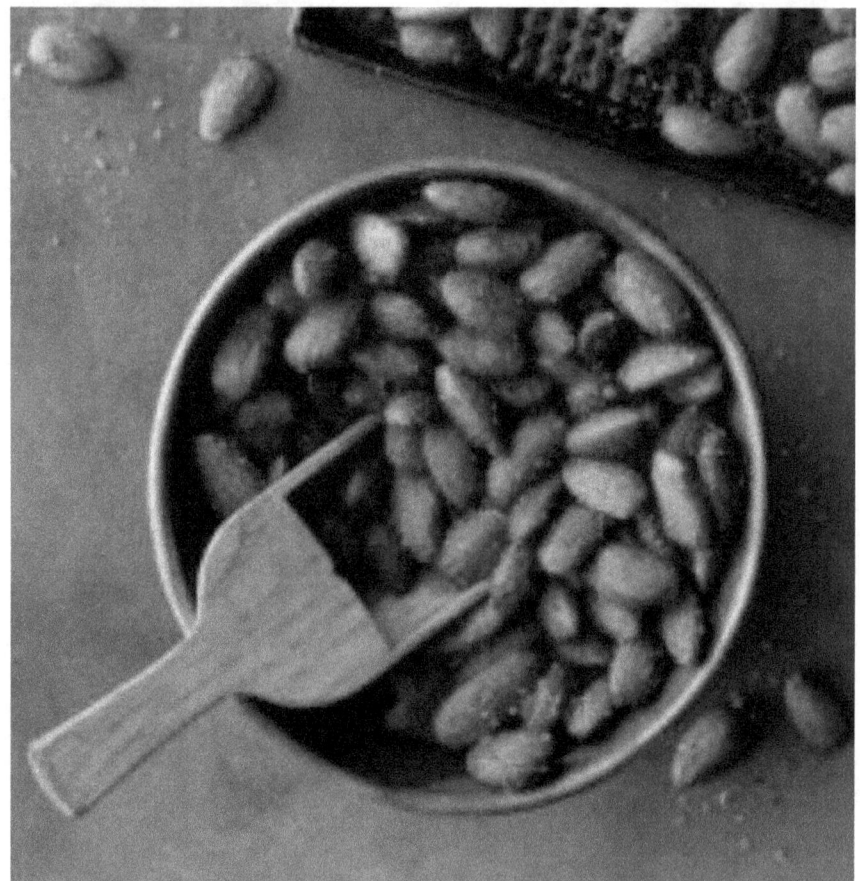

Prep Time: 10 mins.
Cook Time: 30 mins + cooling
Total Time: 40 mins
Servings: 4

Ingredients

- ☐ 1 tablespoon sugar

- ☐ 1-1/2 teaspoons kosher salt

- ☐ 1 teaspoon paprika

- ☐ 1/2 teaspoon ground cinnamon

- ☐ 1/2 teaspoon ground cumin

- ☐ 1/2 teaspoon ground coriander

- ☐ 1/4 teaspoon cayenne pepper

- ☐ 1 large egg white, room temperature

☐ 2-1/2 cups unblanched almonds

Directions

1. Heat oven to 325°. With a small pan, combine the first 7 ingredients. In another little pan, turn the egg white until foamy. Add together almonds; toss to coat. Top up with spice mixture; toss to coat. Spread in a pan on a greased 15x10x1-in. baking skillet. Bake for 30 minutes, stirring every 10 minutes. Spread on paper to cool completely it immediately. Keep in an airtight container.

48. Mimi's Lentil Medley

Prep Time: 15 mins
Cook Time: 25 mins
Total Time: 40 mins
Servings: 8

Ingredients

- ☐ 1 cup dried lentils, rinsed
- ☐ 2 cups water
- ☐ 2 cups sliced fresh mushrooms
- ☐ 1 medium cucumber, cubed
- ☐ 1 medium zucchini, cubed
- ☐ 1 small red onion, chopped
- ☐ 1/2 cup chopped soft sun-dried tomato halves (not packed in oil)
- ☐ 1/2 cup rice vinegar
- ☐ 1/4 cup minced fresh mint
- ☐ 3 tablespoons olive oil
- ☐ 2 teaspoons honey
- ☐ 1 teaspoon dried basil
- ☐ 1 teaspoon dried oregano
- ☐ 4 cups fresh baby spinach, chopped
- ☐ 1 cup (4 ounces) crumbled feta cheese
- ☐ 4 bacon strips, cooked and crumbled, optional

Directions

1. Place lentils in a small saucepan. Add water; bring to a boil. Reduce heat; simmer, covered, 20-25 minutes or until tender. Drain and rinse in cold water.

2. Add it to a large bowl or pan. Include mushrooms, cucumber, zucchini, onion and tomatoes. Stir vinegar, mint, oil, honey, basil and oregano. Drizzle over lentil mixture; toss to coat. Also you can add spinach, cheese and, if desired bacon toss is a combination.

49. Spiced Salmon

Prep Time: 5 mins
Cook Time: 15 mins
Total Time: 20 mins
Servings: 8

Ingredients

- [ ] 2 tablespoons packed brown sugar
- [ ] 1 tablespoon soy sauce
- [ ] 1 tablespoon butter, melted
- [ ] 1 tablespoon olive oil
- [ ] 1/2 teaspoon garlic powder
- [ ] 1/2 teaspoon ground mustard
- [ ] 1/2 teaspoon paprika
- [ ] 1/2 teaspoon pepper
- [ ] 1/4 teaspoon dill weed
- [ ] Dash salt
- [ ] Dash dried tarragon
- [ ] Dash cayenne pepper
- [ ] 1 salmon fillet (2 pounds)

<u>Directions</u>

1. Add all the ingredients except salmon; over look salmon.

2. Add salmon skin offside down, on an oiled grill rack or on a lightly oiled baking pan. Cover the grill with medium heat or broil 4 in. from heat till the fish just begins to flake with a fork, 10-15 minutes.

50. Tomato Green Bean Soup

Prep Time: 10 mins
Cook Time: 35 mins
Total Time: 45 mins
Servings: 2

Ingredients

- ☐ 1 cup chopped onion
- ☐ 1 cup chopped carrots
- ☐ 2 teaspoons butter
- ☐ 6 cups reduced-sodium chicken or vegetable broth
- ☐ 1 pound fresh green beans, cut into 1-inch pieces
- ☐ 1 garlic clove, minced
- ☐ 3 cups diced fresh tomatoes
- ☐ 1/4 cup minced fresh basil or 1 tablespoon dried basil
- ☐ 1/2 teaspoon salt
- ☐ 1/4 teaspoon pepper

Directions

1. With a large saucepan, sauté carrots and onion in butter for about 5 minutes. Stir properly the broth, beans and garlic; add to a boil. Decrease the heat; cover and simmer for 20 minutes or until vegetables are tender.

2. Stir in the tomatoes, basil, salt and pepper. Cover and simmer 5 minutes longer.

51. Cannellini Bean Hummus

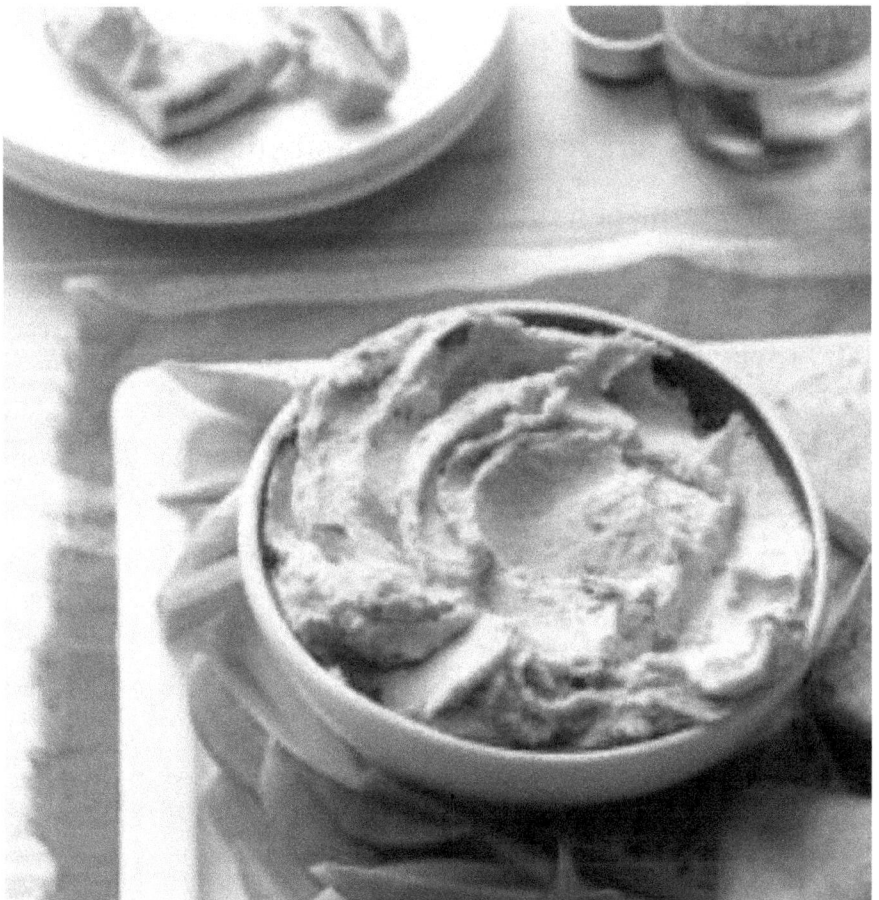

Prep Time: 5 mins
Total Time: 5mins
Servings: 10

Ingredients

- ☐ 2 garlic cloves, peeled
- ☐ 1 can (15 ounces) cannellini beans, rinsed and drained
- ☐ 1/4 cup tahini
- ☐ 3 tablespoons lemon juice
- ☐ 1-1/2 teaspoons ground cumin
- ☐ 1/4 teaspoon salt
- ☐ 1/4 teaspoon crushed red pepper flakes
- ☐ 2 tablespoons minced fresh parsley
- ☐ Pita breads, cut into wedges

☐   Assorted fresh vegetables

Directions

1. Place garlic in a food processor; cover and process until minced. Put the beans, lemon juice, cumin, salt and pepper flakes; cover and process until soften.

2. Change to a small bowl; stir in parsley. Refrigerate until serving. Serve with pita wedges and all kinds of fresh vegetables.

52. Peppered Sole

Prep Time: 10 mins
Cook Time: 15 mins
Total Time: 25 min.
Servings: 4

Ingredients

- ☐ 2 tablespoons butter
- ☐ 2 cups sliced fresh mushrooms
- ☐ 2 garlic cloves, minced
- ☐ 4 sole fillets (4 ounces each)
- ☐ 1/4 teaspoon paprika
- ☐ 1/4 teaspoon lemon-pepper seasoning
- ☐ 1/8 teaspoon cayenne pepper
- ☐ 1 medium tomato, chopped
- ☐ 2 green onions, thinly sliced

Directions

1. Using a large skillet, heat butter over medium-high heat. Put mushrooms; cook and stir until soften. Put garlic; cook 1 minute longer. Place fillets over mushrooms. Sprinkle with paprika, lemon pepper and cayenne.

2. Cover and cook it over medium heat 5-10 minutes or until fish just begins to flake easily with a fork. Sprinkle with tomato and green onions.

53. Portobello Mushrooms Florentine

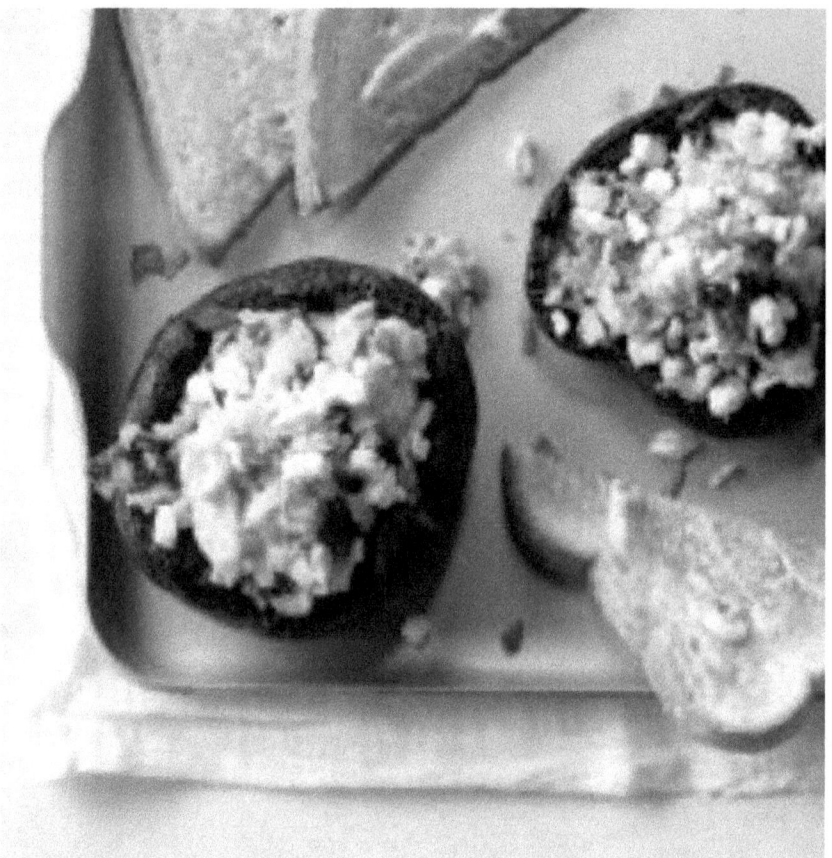

Prep Time: 10 mins
Cook Time: 15 mins
Total Time: 25 min.
Servings : 2

Ingredients

- ☐ 2 large portobello mushrooms, stems removed
- ☐ Cooking spray
- ☐ 1/8 teaspoon garlic salt
- ☐ 1/8 teaspoon pepper
- ☐ 1/2 teaspoon olive oil
- ☐ 1 small onion, chopped
- ☐ 1 cup fresh baby spinach
- ☐ 2 large eggs

- ☐ 1/8 teaspoon salt
- ☐ 1/4 cup crumbled goat or feta cheese
- ☐ Minced fresh basil, optional

Directions

1. Heat oven to 425°. Stir mushrooms with cooking spray; place in a 15x10x1-in. pan, stem side up. Sprinkle with garlic salt and pepper. Bake, uncovered, until tender, about 10 minutes.

2. Before then add nonstick skillet, heat oil over medium-high heat; saute onion until tender. Stir in spinach until wilted.

3. Add together eggs and salt; add to skillet. Cook and stir until eggs are hard and no liquid egg remains; spoon onto mushrooms. Top up with cheese and, if desired, basil.

54. Shrimp Orzo with Feta

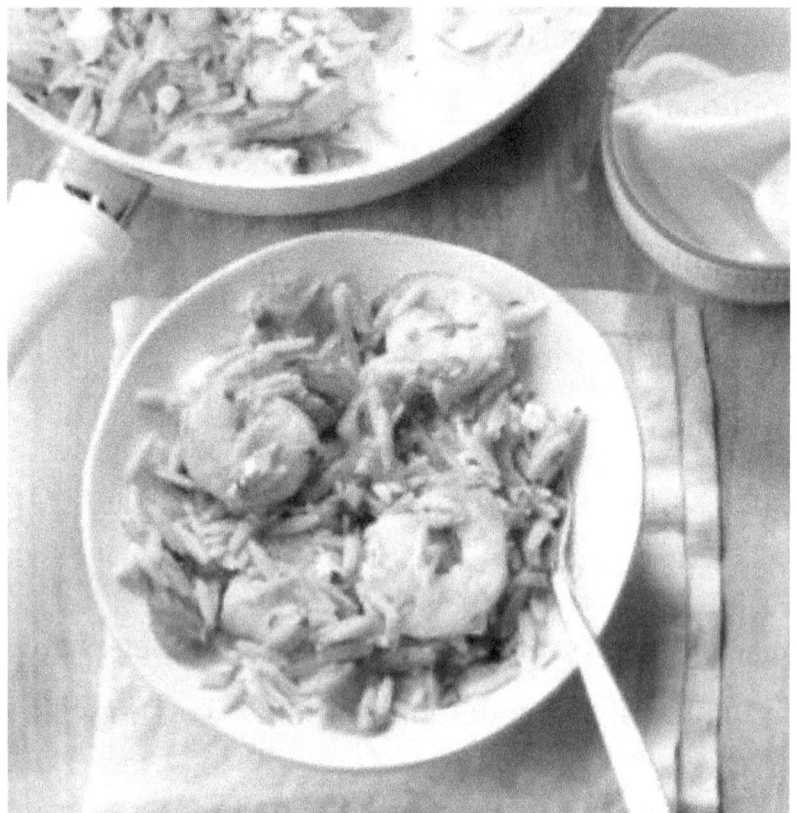

Prep Time: 10 mins
Cook Time: 15 mins
Total Time: 25 min.
Servings : 4

Ingredients

- ☐ 1-1/4 cups uncooked whole wheat orzo pasta
- ☐ 2 tablespoons olive oil
- ☐ 2 garlic cloves, minced
- ☐ 2 medium tomatoes, chopped
- ☐ 2 tablespoons lemon juice
- ☐ 1-1/4 pounds uncooked shrimp (26-30 per pound), peeled and deveined
- ☐ 2 tablespoons minced fresh cilantro
- ☐ 1/4 teaspoon pepper
- ☐ 1/2 cup crumbled feta cheese

Directions

1. Cook orzo according to package directions. Better still, in a large pan, heat oil over medium cooker. Put garlic; cook and stir 1 minute. Include tomatoes and lemon juice. Then to a boil. Stir in shrimp. Decrease the heat; simmer and uncover it until shrimp turn pink, 4-5 minutes.

2. Dry orzo, cilantro and pepper to shrimp together; heat through. Spray with feta cheese.

55. Beef and Blue Cheese Penne with Pesto

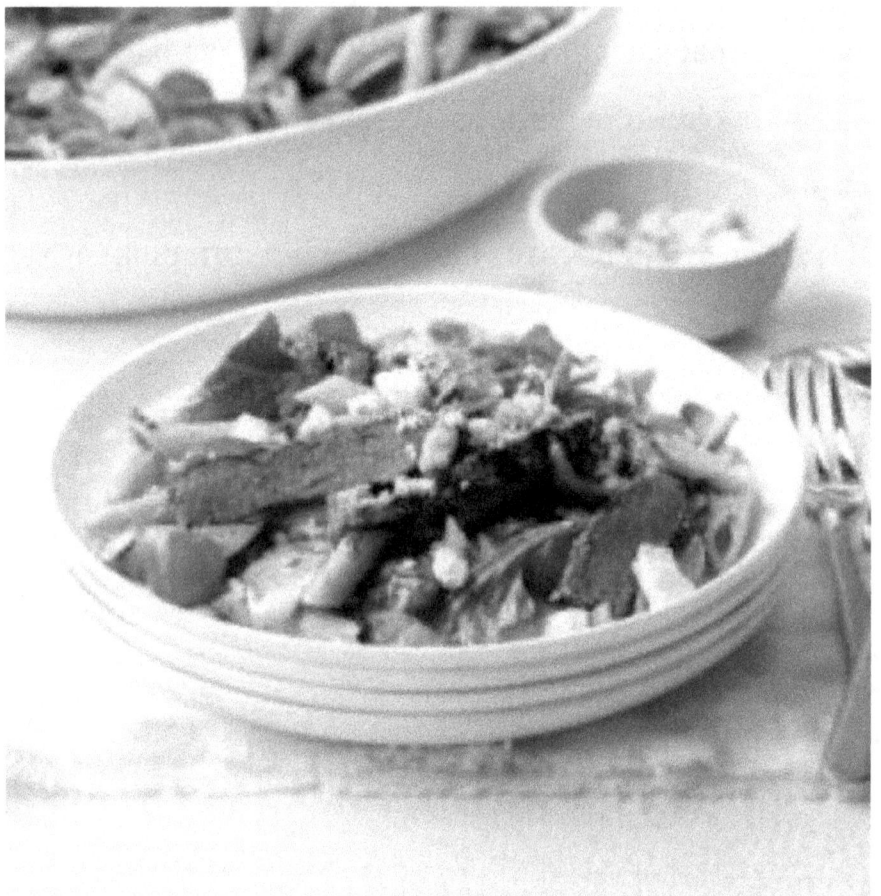

Prep Time: 15 mins
Cook Time: 15 mins
Total Time: 30 mins
Servings : 4

Ingredients

- ☐   2 cups uncooked whole wheat penne pasta
- ☐   2 beef tenderloin steaks (6 ounces each)
- ☐   1/4 teaspoon salt
- ☐   1/4 teaspoon pepper
- ☐   5 ounces fresh baby spinach (about 6 cups), coarsely chopped
- ☐   2 cups grape tomatoes, halved
- ☐   1/3 cup prepared pesto
- ☐   1/4 cup chopped walnuts

☐   1/4 cup crumbled Gorgonzola cheese

Directions

1. Cook pasta according to package directions.

2. Meanwhile, sprinkle steaks with salt and pepper under 5-7 minutes on each side or until meat reaches desired doneness. For medium thermometer should read 135°; medium, 140°; medium-well, 145°).

3. Drain pasta; transfer to a large bowl. Add spinach, tomatoes, pesto and walnuts; toss to coat. Cut steak into thin slices. Serve pasta mixture with beef; sprinkle with cheese.

56. Citrus-Herb Pork Roast

Prep Time: 25 mins

Cook Time: 4 hrs

Total Time: 4 hrs 25 mins

Servings: 8

Ingredients

- ☐ 1 boneless pork sirloin roast (3 to 4 pounds)
- ☐ 1 teaspoon dried oregano
- ☐ 1/2 teaspoon ground ginger
- ☐ 1/2 teaspoon pepper
- ☐ 2 medium onions, cut into thin wedges
- ☐ 1 cup plus 3 tablespoons orange juice, divided
- ☐ 1 tablespoon sugar
- ☐ 1 tablespoon white grapefruit juice
- ☐ 1 tablespoon steak sauce
- ☐ 1 tablespoon reduced-sodium soy sauce
- ☐ 1 teaspoon grated orange zest
- ☐ 1/2 teaspoon salt
- ☐ 3 tablespoons cornstarch
- ☐ Hot cooked egg noodles
- ☐ Minced fresh oregano, optional

Directions

1. Cut roast in a very tiny bowl, mix the oregano, ginger and pepper; rub over pork. in a very massive slippery bowl, coated with cookery spray, brown roast on all sides. Transfer to a 4-qt. slow cooker; add onions.

2. In a very tiny bowl, mix one cup fruit juice, sugar, fruit juice, condiment and soy sauce; pour over prime. cowl and cook on low for 4-5 hours or till meat is tender. Take away meat and onions to a serving platter; keep heat.

3. Skim fat from cookery juices; transfer to a little pan. Add orange rind and salt. Arouse a boil, mix starch and therefore the remaining fruit juice till swish. Step by step stir into the pan. Arouse a boil; cook and stir for two minutes or till thickened. Serve with pork and noodles; if desired, sprinkle with contemporary oregano.

57. Asparagus with Horseradish Dip

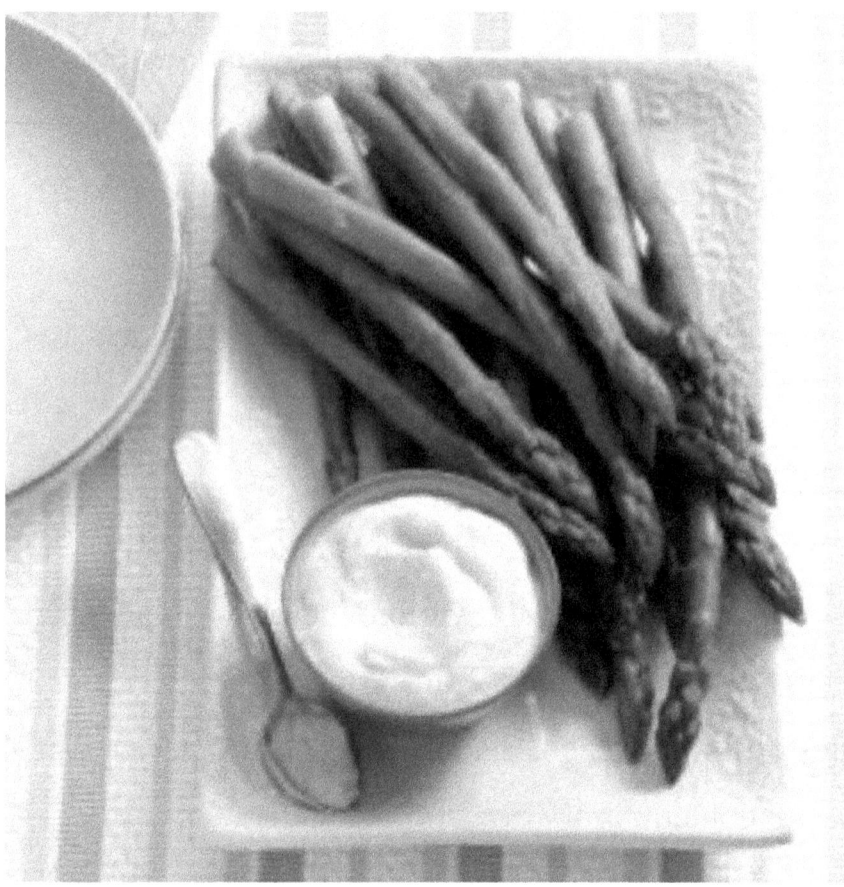

Prep Time: 5 mins
Cook Time: 10 mins
Total Time: 15 min.
Servings: 8

Ingredients

- ☐ 32 fresh asparagus spears (about 2 pounds), trimmed
- ☐ 1 cup reduced-fat mayonnaise
- ☐ 1/4 cup grated Parmesan cheese
- ☐ 1 tablespoon prepared horseradish
- ☐ 1/2 teaspoon Worcestershire sauce

Directions

1. Add asparagus in a steamer basket; place in a large saucepan over 1 in. of water. Bring to a boil; cover and steam until crisp-tender, 2-4 minutes. Drain and immediately place in ice water. Drain and pat dry.

2. With small bowl, add together the left over ingredients. Serve with asparagus.

58. Grilled Tilapia with Pineapple Salsa

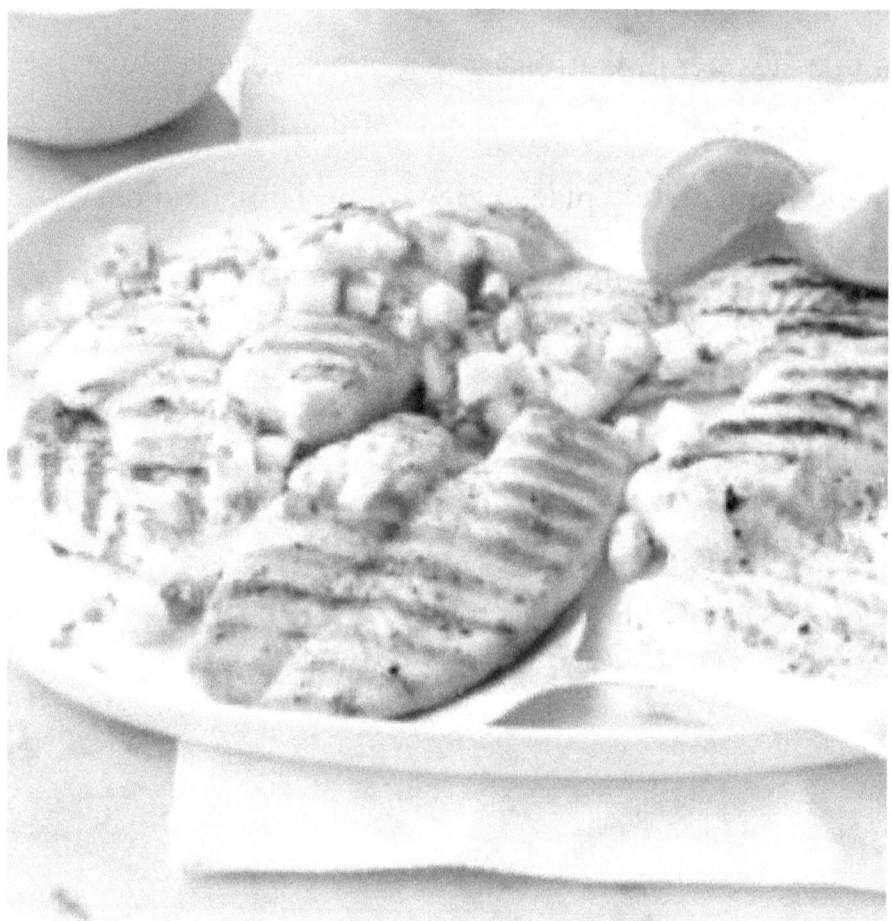

Prep Time: 5 mins
Cook Time: 15 mins
Total Time: 20 mins
Servings: 8

Ingredients

- ☐ 2 cups cubed fresh pineapple
- ☐ 2 green onions, chopped
- ☐ 1/4 cup finely chopped green pepper
- ☐ 1/4 cup minced fresh cilantro
- ☐ 4 teaspoons plus 2 tablespoons lime juice, divided
- ☐ 1/8 teaspoon plus 1/4 teaspoon salt, divided
- ☐ Dash cayenne pepper
- ☐ 1 tablespoon canola oil

- ☐ 8 tilapia fillets (4 ounces each)
- ☐ 1/8 teaspoon pepper

Directions

1. For salsa, add in a small pan, join together pineapple, green onions, green pepper, cilantro, 4 teaspoons lime juice, 1/8 teaspoon salt and cayenne. Refrigerate before serving.

2. Mix oil and remaining lime juice together; drizzle across fillets. swith pepper and remaining salt.

3. Moisten a paper towel with cooking oil; using long-handled tongs, rub on grill spray rack to coat lightly, cover grill fish over medium heat or broil 4 in. from heat 2-3 minutes on each side or until fish just to flake easily with a fork. Serve with salsa if needed.

59. California Quinoa

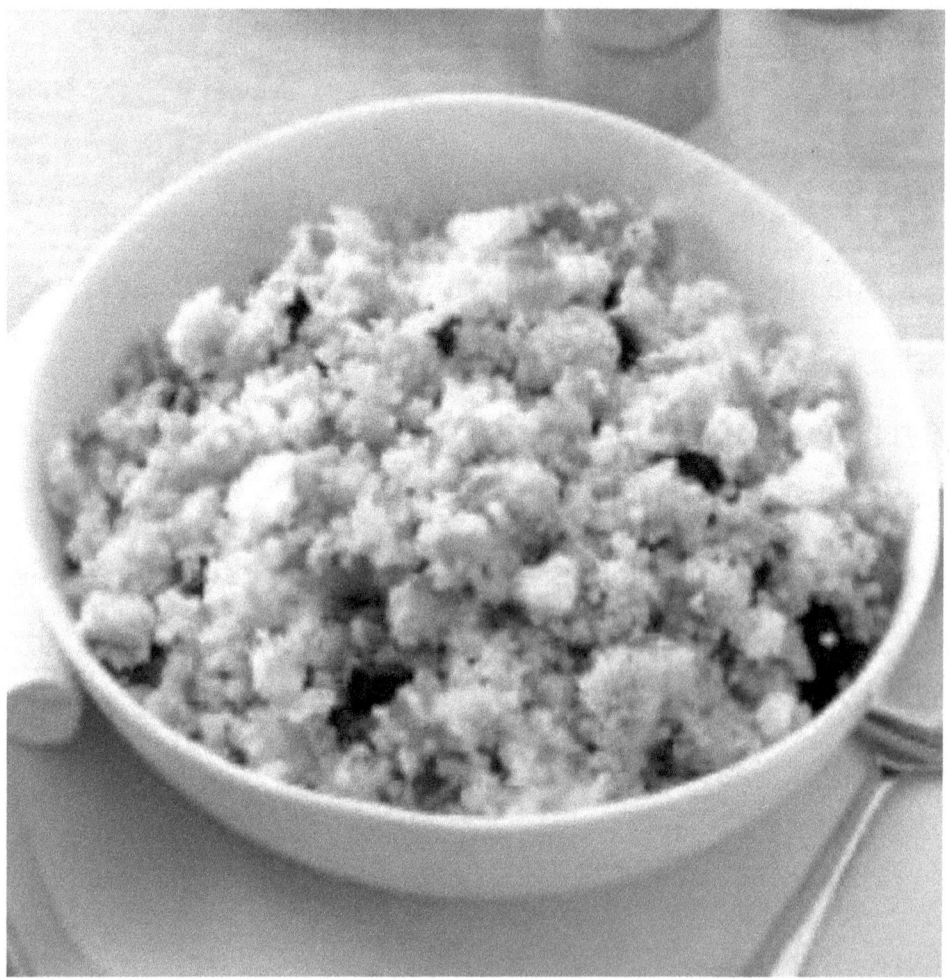

Prep Time: 1o mins
Cook Time: 20 mins
Total Time: 30 min.
Servings: 4

Ingredients

- ☐ 1 tablespoon olive oil
- ☐ 1 cup quinoa, rinsed and well drained
- ☐ 2 garlic cloves, minced
- ☐ 1 medium zucchini, chopped
- ☐ 2 cups water
- ☐ 3/4 cup canned garbanzo beans or chickpeas, rinsed and drained
- ☐ 1 medium tomato, finely chopped

- ☐ 1/2 cup crumbled feta cheese
- ☐ 1/4 cup finely chopped Greek olives
- ☐ 2 tablespoons minced fresh basil
- ☐ 1/4 teaspoon pepper

Directions

1. With a large saucepan, heat oil across medium heat. Include quinoa and garlic; stir and cook until 2-3 minutes or until quinoa is lightly colored. Stir together in zucchini and water; bring to heat. Decrease to heat; simmer, covered, till liquid is dry, 12-15 minutes. Stir in the left over ingredients; heat thoroughly.

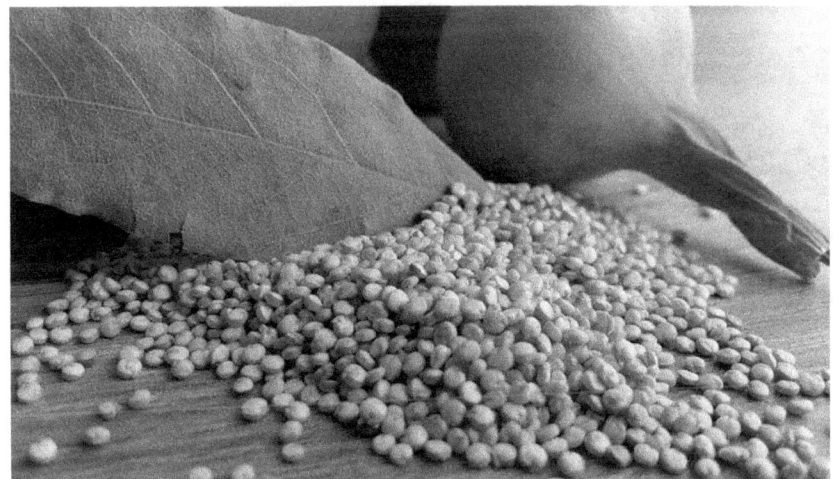

60. Peppered Tuna Kabobs

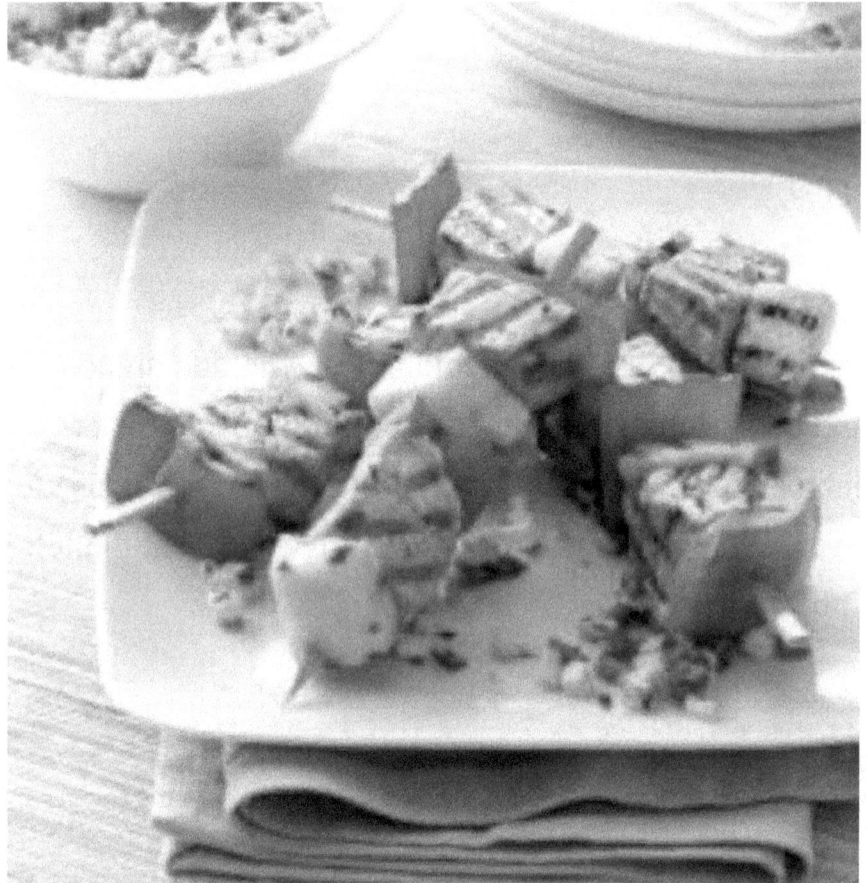

Prep Time: 5 mins
Cook Time: 20 mins
Total Time: 30 min.
Servings :4

Ingredients

- ☐ 1/2 cup frozen corn, thawed
- ☐ 4 green onions, chopped
- ☐ 1 jalapeno pepper, seeded and chopped
- ☐ 2 tablespoons coarsely chopped fresh parsley
- ☐ 2 tablespoons lime juice
- ☐ 1 pound tuna steaks, cut into 1-inch cubes
- ☐ 1 teaspoon coarsely ground pepper
- ☐ 2 large sweet red peppers, cut into 2x1-inch pieces
- ☐ 1 medium mango, peeled and cut into 1-inch cubes

Directions

1. Add salsa, in a little bowl, add the first five ingredients; set aside.

2. Rub tuna with pepper. Use four metal or soaked wooden skewers or thread red peppers, tuna and mango.

3. Use skewers on greased grill rack. Cover it and cook over medium heat, keep turning always, until tuna is slightly turn to pink in center (medium-rare) and peppers are soft, 10-12 minutes. Good with salsa.

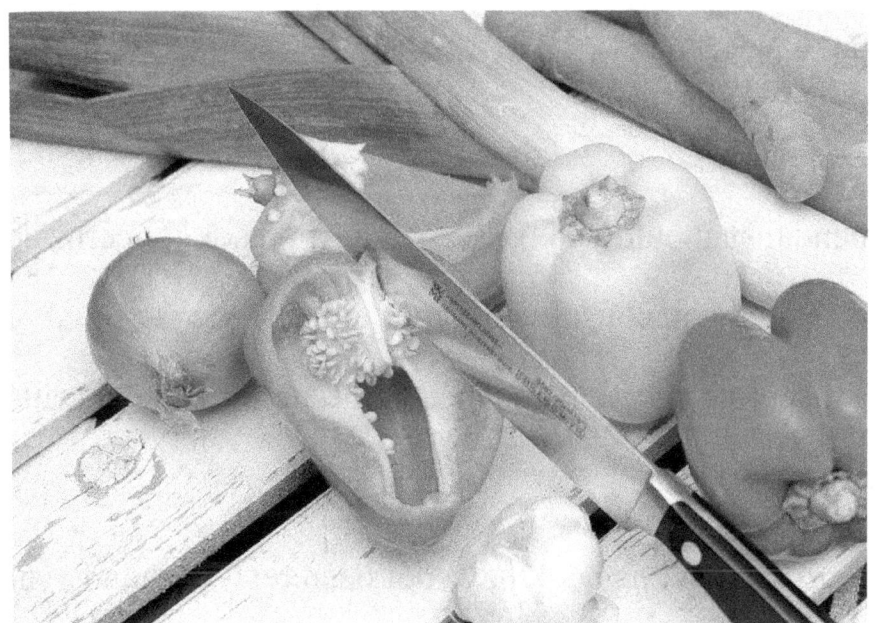

learned from the book. The use of all or any of the information we provide through this book is entirely at your own risk.

Recent developments in the field of medical research may have an impact on the nutritional, health, and fitness information discussed in this book. We are giving no assurance that the information contained in this book will always reflect the latest developments or findings in the field.

We believe that the information we provide in this book is accurate at the time of writing. The content of this book is based on thorough research and our better judgment. However, just like any material, it may become obsolete over time.

The information in this book may contain some technical errors or inaccuracies and may be updated or changed without notice.

Users agree that access and use of all information in the book are at their own risk. We do not assume any liability for any information contained herein.

When you think that you are experiencing a health or medical emergency, do not hesitate to call your health care professional right away.

CONCLUSION

The DASH diet recommends increased consumption of fruits, vegetables, low-fat dairy, whole grains, poultry, fish, and nuts while limiting the intake of red meat and added sugars. It is relatively low in total fat, saturated fat (6%), and sodium (2300 mg/day). There is substantial evidence that the DASH diet consistently reduces blood pressure. Different variations of the DASH diet have been examined. While the findings indicate that these DASH-style diets are cardio protective, the extent of their beneficial impact on different cardiovascular risk factors varies.

The DASH diet is a healthfully based way to deal with and control hypertension. The diet has been tried in a few clinical preliminaries and has been appeared to bring down cholesterol, saturated fats, and blood pressure. The DASH diet has been prescribed as the best diet to help individuals who might want to lose or keep up a solid weight and lower the blood pressure. The key actuality is that this diet should be elevated to patients. Other than doctors, the two nurses and drug specialists assume a key job in instructing patients about the benefits of this diet. Only preceding release, nurses are in a prime situation to educate all patients and their families about the DASH diet and its benefits. So also, when patients visit a drug store, the drug specialist ought to educate the patient about the DASH diet. The most significant component of the DASH diet is it requires an adjustment in the way of life and embrace a sound method to eat. Also, patients ought to be asked to quit smoking, swear off liquor and alcohol and do some kind of physical activities all the time.

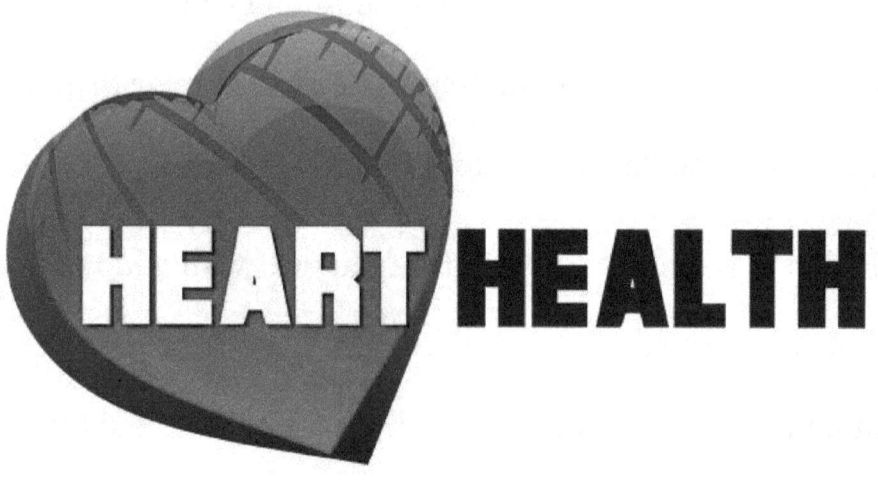

CPSIA information can be obtained
at www.ICGtesting.com
Printed in the USA
BVHW050534150521
607370BV00005B/422